Pulmonary Reactions to Coal Dust

A REVIEW OF U. S. EXPERIENCE

ENVIRONMENTAL SCIENCES

An Interdisciplinary Monograph Series

EDITORS

DOUGLAS H. K. LEE
National Institute of
Environmental Health Sciences
Research Triangle Park
North Carolina

E. WENDELL HEWSON
Department of
Atmospheric Science
Oregon State University
Corvallis, Oregon

DANIEL OKUN
University of North Carolina
Department of Environmental
Sciences and Engineering
Chapel Hill, North Carolina

PULMONARY REACTIONS TO COAL DUST

A REVIEW OF U. S. EXPERIENCE

Edited by MARCUS M. KEY

DIRECTOR
BUREAU OF OCCUPATIONAL SAFETY AND HEALTH
U. S. DEPARTMENT OF HEALTH, EDUCATION AND WELFARE
ROCKVILLE, MARYLAND

LORIN E. KERR

DIRECTOR
DEPARTMENT OF OCCUPATIONAL HEALTH
UNITED MINE WORKERS OF AMERICA
WASHINGTON, D. C.

MERLE BUNDY

MEDICAL DIRECTOR
U. S. STEEL CORPORATION
PITTSBURGH, PENNSYLVANIA

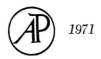 *1971*

ACADEMIC PRESS   New York and London

ACADEMIC PRESS, INC.
111 Fifth Avenue, New York, New York 10003

United Kingdom Edition published by
ACADEMIC PRESS, INC. (LONDON) LTD.
Berkeley Square House, London W1X 6BA

LIBRARY OF CONGRESS CATALOG CARD NUMBER: 74-159612

PRINTED IN THE UNITED STATES OF AMERICA

Contents

Part 2   CLINICAL CHARACTERISTICS

Chapter 3.   Extent and Distribution of Respiratory Effects

William S. Lainhart and W. Keith C. Morgan

Chapter 4.   Symptomatology

Murray B. Hunter

Part 3   TREATMENT AND CONTROL

Chapter 10.   Etiology

Douglas H. K. Lee

Chapter 11.   Treatment

Leon Cander

Chapter 12.   Investigations in Progress

Biomedical

W. Keith C. Morgan and Earle P. Shoub

Instrumentation

Jeremiah R. Lynch

List of Contributors

Numbers in parentheses indicate the pages on which the authors' contributions begin.

LEONARD J. BRISTOL, M.D. (111), Director, Silicosis Control Unit, Medical Research Laboratories, Trudeau Institute, Incorporated, Saranac Lake, New York

LEON CANDER, M.D. (197), Professor and Chairman, Department of Physiology and Medicine, The University of Texas Medical School at San Antonio, Texas

NICHOLAS L. FANNICK (13), Industrial Hygienist, Health Division, Coal Mine Health and Safety, Bureau of Mines, Department of the Interior, Washington, D. C.

BENJAMIN FELSON, M.D., F.C.C.P. (111), Professor and Director, Radiology Department, University of Cincinnati, Cincinnati, Ohio

MURRAY B. HUNTER, M.D. (57), Fairmont Clinic, Fairmont, West Virginia

GEORGE JACOBSON, M.D. (111), Professor and Chairman, Radiology Department, University of Southern California, Los Angeles, California

WILLIAM S. LAINHART, M.D. (29, 111), Deputy Director, Division of Epidemiology and Special Services, Bureau of Occupational Safety and Health, Department of Health, Education and Welfare, Cincinnati, Ohio

N. LeRoy Lapp, M.D. (153), Appalachian Laboratory for Occupational Respiratory Diseases, Bureau of Occupational Safety and Health, Department of Health, Education and Welfare, West Virginia University Medical Center, Morgantown, West Virginia

Douglas H. K. Lee, M.D. (1, 189), National Institute of Environmental Health Sciences, National Institutes of Health, Department of Health, Education and Welfare, Research Triangle Park, North Carolina

Jeremiah R. Lynch (212), Bureau of Occupational Safety and Health, Department of Health, Education and Welfare, Cincinnati, Ohio

W. Keith C. Morgan, M.D. (29, 205), Chief, Appalachian Laboratory for Occupational Respiratory Diseases, Morgantown, West Virginia

Richard L. Naeye, M.D. (93), Department of Pathology, M. S. Hershey Medical Center, Hershey, Pennsylvania

Eugene P. Pendergrass, M.D. (111), Emeritus Professor of Radiology, Hospital of the University of Pennsylvania, Philadelphia, Pennsylvania

R. W. Penman, M.D. (181), Professor of Medicine, Director, Pulmonary Division, University of Kentucky Medical Center, Lexington, Kentucky

Donald P. Schlick (13), Chief, Health Division, Coal Mine Health and Safety, Bureau of Mines, Department of the Interior, Washington, D. C.

Earle P. Shoub (205), Deputy Chief, Appalachian Laboratory for Occupational Respiratory Diseases, Morgantown, West Virginia

Anthony Seaton, M.D. (153), Appalachian Laboratory for Occupational Respiratory Diseases, Bureau of Occupational Safety and Health, Department of Health, Education and Welfare, West Virginia University Medical Center, Morgantown, West Virginia

John P. Wyatt, M.D. (71), Department of Pathology, Faculty of Medicine, University of Manitoba, Winnipeg, Canada

Preface

The health of the coal miner, particularly the frequency of respiratory disorders in miners and former miners, has long been a matter of concern to physicians practicing in coal fields in the United States. That coal dust could play a specific role in the etiology of the miner's respiratory troubles, however, long went unacknowledged. Attention had been dramatically focused on the devastating effects of silica dust, but there was little silica in coal dust, so that the idea of a true dust disease, or pneumoconiosis, did not find ready favor.

Several years passed before coal workers' pneumoconiosis was accorded the recognition in this country that it had received in 1942 in Britain. When finally the acknowledgment was made, the excellent investigative work done in that country loomed so large that there seemed little point in pursuing the matter much further. The point had been made that coal dust could produce pneumoconiotic changes, and the implications for control seemed clear. All that was needed was a good measure of the extent to which the condition prevailed here so that the amount of control required could be gauged.

As the surveys went forward, however, doubts began to arise as to whether what is seen in the United States coal fields is exactly the same as that seen in Britain. Tuberculosis is less prevalent here, but progressive massive fibrosis develops about as readily. Rank of coal, the geological nature of the seams, and various other features are far from identical in the two locations. Evidence mounted that investigators might not be talking about exactly the same thing in the two countries and that the implications for control might be different.

In the fall of 1969 it was felt that prevailing opinions in this country should be gathered into a book which would (a) establish an American view of the disease picture; (b) provide a reference for legislative and control purposes; (c) promote interaction between medical, scientific, and administrative aspects; and (d) provide a point of departure for international discussions. For the first time, in this biomedically oriented book, American views and experience on most aspects of the disease have been brought together for comparison with each other and with those in other countries. It will be clear to the reader that there is still room for difference of opinion on the exact nature and progress of the disease picture and even on the extent to which coal dust as such enters into the essential etiology. But the trend is fairly clear, with coal dust playing a variable but significant role as a clinical entity that is markedly pleomorphic. It would be premature to seek greater consensus at this time, but the interaction now initiated will certainly lead to better understanding and agreement.

It is gratifying to note the way in which a medicoscientific community has grown up around the problem and also the way in which this cooperation enters into all phases of the mining industry as evidenced by the affiliations of the three book editors. We are happy to be able to include such a volume in the Environmental Sciences Series and note that the timing is particularly appropriate in view of the increasing medical and sociological interest in the welfare of coal miners.

The opinions expressed by the contributors in this book are those of the individuals concerned and do not necessarily reflect those of the organizations to which they belong.

DOUGLAS H. K. LEE
DANIEL A. OKUN
E. WENDELL HEWSON

Pulmonary Reactions to Coal Dust

A REVIEW OF U. S. EXPERIENCE

PART 1
BACKGROUND

1

Historical Aspects

Douglas H. K. Lee

To those interested in the development and dissemination of ideas, the story of coal workers' pneumoconiosis (CWP) in the United States, as compared with that in Britain, must present many enigmas—enigmas no less remarkable for their repetition in the story of byssinosis.

Whatever the explanation offered—easier communication in a smaller community; longer experience with coal mining; greater familiarity with the hazards of coal mining; widespread personal experience of smog and its relation to coal fires; a sharper, because delayed, rise of social consciousness—the fact remains that in Britain recognition of the syndrome and attention to its prevention antedated their counterparts in the United States by some 30 years.

The general tardiness of coal mine legislation in this country is revealed by the following summary:

1865: Bill is introduced to create "Federal Mining Bureau"—not passed.
1910: Bureau of Mines is established, but specifically denied right of inspection.
1941: Bureau of Mines is granted authority to inspect, but it is not given authority to establish or enforce safety codes (Title I Federal Coal Mine Safety Act).
1946: Federal Mine Safety Code for Bituminous Coal and Lignite Mines is issued by the Director, Bureau of Mines (agreement between Secretary of the Interior and the United Mine Workers of America) and included in the 1946 (Krug–Lewis) UMWA Wage Agreement.
1947: Congress requests coal mine operators and State Agencies to report compliance with the Federal Mine Safety Code. Thirty-three percent compliance is reported.
1952: Title II of the Federal Coal Mine Safety Act is passed. All mines

employing 15 or more persons underground must comply with the Act. Enforcement is limited to issuing orders of withdrawal for imminent danger or for failure to abate violations within a reasonable time.

1966: Amendments to 1952 law. Mines employing under 15 employees are included under 1952 Act; stronger regulatory powers are given to Bureau of Mines, such as the provision permitting the closing of a mine or section of a mine because of an unwarrantable failure to correct a dangerous condition.

1969: Federal Coal Mine Health and Safety Act is passed. In this Act the hazards of pneumoconiosis are, for the first time, given prominence, in addition to those of accidents.*

As a source of power essential to the industrial revolution, coal assumed an importance in the eighteenth and early nineteenth centuries seldom achieved by a single commodity. As mine workings increased in depth and complexity, the ventilation, which had improved at first, became more difficult and the dust content rose to very high levels, restricted only by the absolute necessity of keeping dust and methane gas down to levels at which explosion hazards were eliminated, or at least rendered sufficiently infrequent.

Meikeljohn (2, 3) and Rosen (4) indicate that the outstanding blackness of coal miners' lungs had been recognized in Britain by 1813, and the association of a respiratory disease was recognized by 1833. But there the matter seems to have rested. The improvement made for a variety of reasons in mine ventilation apparently satisfied the collective conscience. "Miners' asthma" was well known, but after all, in the murky environment of industrial Britain, miners were not the only ones with respiratory woes.

Importance Attached to Silica

The rapid rise of mining for gold and other minerals at the turn of the century drew attention to a new hazard—that of silica dust. Its importance as a determinant of severe lung disease (miners' phthisis) came into sharp focus. South African and Australian mining experience impressed British physicians. Attention was similarly directed to silica and silicosis in the United States by the afflictions of granite and sandstone cutters, by pulmonary disease developing in hard-rock miners, and by the disastrous affair of the Gauley tunnel. Here, then, appeared to be the key. To the extent that undue respiratory disease occurred in coal miners, it was attributable to associated silica in the country rock—an explanation so logical that further investigation seemed superfluous.

---

* The above summary was prepared from evidence presented to the U. S. Senate Committee on Labor and Public Welfare, 17 September 1969 (1) after discussion with Lorin Kerr (UMWA) and a representative of the U. S. Bureau of Mines.

In the United States this attitude was reinforced, if anything, by the results of the first systematic investigation of coal miners over the period 1928–1931. The investigation was conducted in the anthracite mines of Pennsylvania in which the silica content is relatively high, and the term "anthracosilicosis" was coined for the condition found in the miners' lungs. The results indicated (5–8):

The prevalence of anthracosilicosis among the entire group of employees was found to be about 23%. Among all except rockworkers, less than 2% of the men developed anthracosilicosis when the duration of employment was less than 15 years, regardless of the amount of dust in the air. Among men exposed for 15–24 years to dust containing less than 5% free silica, 14% of those who had worked where the average dust count was 100–199 million particles/ft^3, 29% of those exposed to 200–299 million particles, and 58% of the men who had worked for this period in more than 300 million particles/ft^3 developed anthracosilicosis.

Among men working for more than 25 years in dust containing less than 5% free silica, the proportion of persons found with anthracosilicosis under different concentrations of dust was as follows: 5–99 million particles/ft^3, 7%; 100–199 million particles/ft^3, 54%; 200–299 million particles/ft^3, 71%; 300 or more million particles/ft^3, 89%.

With the exception of miners, their helpers, and rockworkers, about 25% of all of the men employed underground developed anthracosilicosis after a working period of more than 25 years. This group was exposed to dust having a quartz content of about 13%.

The prevalence of anthracosilicosis among rockworkers who had been exposed to dust, of which about 35% was free silica, varied from 10% among those who had worked in concentrations of less than 200 million particles/ft^3 for less than 15 years to 92% among those rockworkers who had been employed for more than 25 years in dust concentrations exceeding 300 million particles/ft^3.

The prevalence of pulmonary tuberculosis among the hard-coal mining employees at ages below 35 was slightly less than that found through studies of tuberculosis among male adults in the general population of the country. In the age group 35–44, however, the prevalence of tuberculosis was about twice; at age 45–54, about 5 times; and for the ages above 55, it was about 10 times the rate found in the general population.

Mortality from respiratory diseases was found to be much greater among anthracite workers than in the general adult male population of the country. The data indicated that underground work in the absence of dust did not predispose to fatal attacks of respiratory disease.

The correlations between exposure to dust and the evidence of constitutional changes left little doubt as to the etiological significance of the dust in the air breathed. Like correlations were found between the silica exposure and the extent of pulmonary changes.

In an investigation carried out in 1938–1939 in Utah, the United States Public Health Service found the incidence of anthracosilicosis among 346 underground bituminous-coal miners to be 4.6%.

Other Etiological Factors Considered

Not everyone, however, accepted the simple explanation. Even before the turn of the century, the idea was being expressed in Britain that coal miners suffered from a somewhat unusual form of chest disease. A compromise concept was developed that coal dust whose elimination from the lung was blocked by reaction to silica could produce disease (9). By 1928 Collis and Gilchrist had shown (10, 11) that British coal trimmers (an occupational category now fortunately extinct) showed pneumoconiotic changes in their lungs, even though the coal that they shovelled had been washed relatively free of country rock. The coal could still have contained some silica, but these workers' lungs yielded no abnormal quantities of silica at autopsy. By 1934, according to Hunter (12), British physicians were beginning to accept coal dust as a cause of a slowly progressive and fatal disease.

Out of the argument development began in 1936 of a systematic study of bituminous-coal miners by the Committee on Industrial Pulmonary Diseases of the Medical Research Council. In its 1942 report (13) the term "coal workers' pneumoconiosis" was introduced. This term, which avoids any implication about the etiological role of any silica that may be present, is now in general use. The Pneumoconiosis Research Unit, set up by the Medical Research Council in South Wales in 1945, has continued to advance our knowledge of the disease (14) and has confirmed the value of control measures introduced by the National Coal Board. In 1950 the International Labour Office (15) adopted a standard method of classifying radiographic changes developed by British workers.

Meanwhile, concepts of respiratory disease in coal miners continued along classical lines in the United States. A significant incidence of silicosis in anthracite miners was generally accepted after the 1936 report of Dreessen and Jones (8). But in 1933 Brundage (16) had shown that deaths from all respiratory diseases were about 25% higher than normal in bituminous miners and 50% higher in anthracite miners, and in 1941 Clarke and Moffet (17) reported finding a tendency to silicosis and "presilicosis" in Appalachian bituminous-coal miners. In the following year, Public Health Service investigators reported much the same for bituminous coal miners in Utah (18), and Jones (19) indicated that it was not a rare disease in bituminous coal miners. By 1949 the role of silica in the lung disease of soft as well as of hard coal miners was well accepted, although the paper of Gordon *et al.* (20) made some concession to the role of carbon in defining anthracosilicosis as "the condition of progressive pulmonary fibrosis with conglomeration of nodules in the advanced stages, caused by the inhalation of carbon and silica, and characterized clinically by dyspnea, with varying degrees of disability." The British term *coal workers' pneumoconiosis* was reserved for "bizarre and varied lesions of pulmonary fibrosis, with emphysema, marked areas of conglomeration, and distension of the bronchi" (21). The survey of hospitalized cases by Gordon *et al.* (20) was also notable for including some tests of pulmonary function in addition to radiographs.

Slowly, however, an accumulation of observations began to erode the preoccupation with silica as the sole culprit. The fact that disease was present in bituminous as well as in anthracite miners, whereas the silica content of the rock was different, was a telling point. Public health workers generally became convinced that coal dust itself was pathogenic, but still found themselves up against the argument that if there is no silica, then there can be no disease. This, coupled with the older belief that coal miners with lung disease are simply people with lung disease who happen to be coal miners, presented a formidable tradition. Requests for funds to elicit evidence on the incidence of disease were apt to be met with demands that evidence be produced to justify the expenditure.

By the early fifties some evidence had accumulated that a large part of the morbidity pattern of bituminous-coal miners was due to chest disease (22, 23). In 1954 the U. S. Public Health Service published a bibliography of British and American investigations (24). In 1957 Levin and Hunter (25) reported pneumoconiosis, identical with that seen in British coal miners, in a small group of Ohio miners. Lieben and others (26–29) over the period 1959–1961 showed that roentgenographic evidence of pneumoconiosis was present in a high percentage (11–29) of bituminous-coal miners in central and western Pennsylvania. The relative contributions of silica and coal dust to the causation remained obscure, however, because of technical inadequacies in environmental sampling. Stoeckle *et al.* (30) in 1961 pointed out the multiplicity of factors that can enter into the etiology of respiratory disease in soft-coal miners.

Appalachian Studies and Legislation

By the middle of 1962 the increasing weight of evidence had made itself felt at Congressional levels. Senator Robert C. Byrd (D., W. Va.)

introduced a line of questioning in the appropriation hearings on the Division of Occupational Health (31) which indicated the need for an assessment of respiratory disease in coal miners and which led to the insertion in the record of the facilities required. Funding, modest at first but later augmented, followed. On 3 January 1963, a U. S. Public Health Service field team began a carefully designed survey in the Appalachian bituminous coal fields to determine the prevalence and nature of respiratory disorders as judged by symptomatology, chest radiography, and pulmonary function tests. In addition to the working miners, the survey included men who had, for ill health or other reasons, given up coal mining. The study was extended to include a sampling of respiratory conditions in miners' wives, as well as in nonminers, in two communities embracing both mining and nonmining occupations.

The results of this study, involving 2549 working and 1191 nonworking miners, were made available informally to Congressional and other interested parties and in summarized form in technical publications (32, 33), but a full-fledged, formal report was not published until June 1969 (21). Radiographic evidence of pneumoconiosis was found in about 9% of working miners and in about 18% of former miners.

In 1967 the Pennsylvania Department of Public Health reported that 19,175 coal miners had radiographic evidence of the disease and 23,768 more were disabled by it (34).

As the information became known, pressure for the introduction of preventive measures and for the compensation of men disabled by the disease mounted. Some improvement in compensation provisions had been introduced by State Legislatures, but preventive measures lagged. Two events brought matters to a head. One was a disastrous mine accident at Farmington, W. Va., on 20 November 1968, which claimed the lives of 78 miners and led to vehement criticism of mine safety practices. The other was the public outcry against black lung disease made by labor groups, Ralph Nader, and others.

The coal miners of West Virginia took time out in March 1969 to exert pressure on the government of that State for protective legislation and improvement in compensation laws. As a result, the Workmen's Compensation Law, State of West Virginia, Chapter 23, was amended (35) as of 1 July 1970 to extend to occupational pneumoconiosis in general the provisions formerly restricted to silicosis alone, with corresponding changes in the name and function of the Board which examines claims made under the Act. Doubtless to avoid any future tribulations of medical semantics, *occupational pneumoconiosis* is defined as "a disease of the lungs caused by the inhalation of minute particles of dust over a period of time due to causes and conditions arising out of and in the course of the employment." It includes, but is not limited to "such diseases as silicosis, anthracosilicosis, coal worker's pneumoconiosis, commonly known as black lung or miner's asthma, silicotuberculosis (silicosis accompanied by active tuberculosis of the lungs), coal worker's pneumoconiosis accompanied by active tuberculosis of the lungs, asbestosis, siderosis, anthrax, and any and all other dust diseases of the lungs and conditions and diseases caused by occupational pneumoconiosis which are not specifically designated herein meeting the definition of occupational pneumoconiosis set forth in the immediately preceding sentence."

Federal Legislation

The criticisms and demonstrations, just and unjust, also helped set the stage for the introduction and ultimate enactment of the Federal Coal Mine Health and Safety Act (Public Law 91-173) on 30 December 1969. This Act provides *inter alia* for:

> Mandatory health standards for protection of life and prevention of occupational disease
>
> Governmental inspections and investigations with right of entry
>
> Power to order withdrawal of an area from operations, abatement orders, and penalties for noncompliance
>
> Dust standards of 3 mg/m³, to be lowered after 3 years to 2 mg/m³
>
> Periodic medical examination of miners, including chest radiographs at stipulated intervals
>
> Transfer of affected miners to less dusty areas
>
> Autopsies of deceased miners
>
> Benefits for total disability from pneumoconiosis, and to widows of miners who die from the disease
>
> Studies, research, experiments, and demonstrations
>
> Assistance to states

Specifications for the medical examinations required under the Act were published in the Federal Register on 14 August 1970.

As might be expected, there are those who feel that the provisions are too restrictive and hard to meet, while others point out inadequacies. Time will show what modifications, amplifications, or additions may be necessary. For the present, the Act can be hailed as an indication that the United States is at last giving the attention to the health and safety of its coal miners that modern medicine and social consciousness demand.

Research

It should be pointed out, of course, that medicine and medical science were not totally inactive while legal developments were in gestation.

They can take some satisfaction in having provided the evidence, if not the final thrust, that brought the legislation into being. In 1964 Enterline showed that the death rates for coal miners are nearly twice those for all working men in the United States (36), and over the last 10 years there has been extensive research aimed at elucidating the real nature of respiratory disease in coal miners, its basic pathology, its relationship to nonspecific as well as to other pneumoconiotic respiratory diseases, and the possible synergistic role of factors other than dust (37).

Within the Public Health Service, research had its focal point, first (1963) in the United Mine Workers Memorial Hospital at Beckley, W. Va., and later (1966) in the Appalachian Laboratory for Occupational Respiratory Diseases (ALFORD) at Morgantown, W. Va., which was set up by the Division of Occupational Health in collaboration with the Medical School of the University of West Virginia. The level of funding for these activities has remained near the one million dollar mark, with two and three quarter million added in 1970 for DHEW's part in the implementation of the Federal Coal Mine Health and Safety Act. Research on coal workers' pneumoconiosis continued at several academic centers, partially supported by grants from the U. S. Public Health Service. Numerous investigations of other pneumoconiotic conditions, of particle distribution in respired air, and of general pulmonary physiology and pathology provided wider understanding of the more specific conditions in coal workers. The U. S. Public Health Service panel of radiological consultants helped to develop the UICC/Cincinnati classification of the pneumoconiosis in 1968 (38), which became the extended form of the revised (1968) ILO classification (39).

Illustrative of the many meetings and conferences which have tried recently to bring together the various pieces of evidence are Pennsylvania Governor's Conference on Pneumoconiosis, 1964 (40); Public Health Service Conference on CWP, Morgantown, 1965; Panel Discussion, National Institute of Environmental Health Sciences, 17 June 1969 (41); International Conference on CWP, Spindletop Research Inc., 10–12 September 1969 (42, 43); Symposium on Respirable Coal Mine Dust, Department of the Interior and others, 3–4 November 1969 (44); National Conference of Medicine and the Federal Coal Mine Health and Safety Act of 1969, University of California School of Public Health and Howard University College of Medicine, Washington, D. C., 15–18 June 1970 (45).

The present volume, planned as a preliminary to an International Conference on Coal Workers' Pneumoconiosis, called by the New York Academy of Sciences for the fall of 1971, presents the picture of the disease as currently seen in the United States. Comparison with the views prevailing in Britain and elsewhere will undoubtedly reveal differences.

Some of the differences will simply represent insufficient knowledge, others will prove to be due to differences in coal or rock composition, mining practices, living conditions, or even ethnic backgrounds. Further exploration of these differences will refine knowledge and suggest improved preventive methods. History will not stand still.

ACKNOWLEDGMENTS

The author is greatly indebted to the three editors for the abundance of information that they have provided. He is particularly obliged to Mr. Henry N. Doyle, formerly an Associate Director of the Division of Occupational Health, for permission to draw heavily on the historical information that he gives in the Bureau publication, "Pneumoconiosis in Appalachian Bituminous Coal Miners" (21). The author's dependence upon Rosen's comprehensive text (4) and Meiklejohn's series of three historical papers (2, 3) will have been clearly recognized by the reader.

REFERENCES

1. Williams, H. A. (1969). "Federal Coal Mine Health and Safety Act of 1969." *U. S. Senate Rep.* 91, p. 411.
2. Meiklejohn, A. (1951). *Brit. J. Ind. Med.* 8, 127.
3. Meiklejohn, A. (1952). *Brit. J. Ind. Med.* 9, 93, 208.
4. Rosen, G. (1943). "History of Miners' Diseases." Schuman, New York.
5. Office of Industrial Hygiene and Sanitation (1933). *U. S. Pub. Health Bull.* 208.
6. Sayers, R. R., *et al.* (1934). *Pa. Dept. Labor Ind., Spec. Bull.* 41.
7. Sayers, R. R., *et al.* (1935). *U. S. Pub. Health Bull.* 221.
8. Dreessen, W. C., and Jones, R. R. (1936). *J. Amer. Med. Ass.* **107**, 1179.
9. Cummins, S. L. (1927). *J. Pathol. Bacteriol.* **30**, 615.
10. Collis, E. L., and Gilchrist, J. C. (1928). *J. Ind. Hyg.* **10**, 101.
11. Gough, J. (1940). *J. Pathol. Bacteriol.* **51**, 277.
12. Hunter, D. (1959). "Health in Industry." Penguin, Middlesex, England.
13. Committee on Industrial Pulmonary Disease (1942, 1943). *Med. Res. Counc. Gt. Brit. Spec. Rep. Ser.* 243, 244.
14. Fletcher, C. M., and Gough, J. (1950). *Brit. Med. Bull.* **7**, 42.
15. International Labour Office (1953). "Suggested International Scheme for the Classification of Radiographs in Some of the Pneumoconioses." *Proc. 3rd Int. Conf. Pneumoconiosis, Geneva,* Vol. I, p. 130.
16. Brundage, D. K. (1933). *U. S. Pub. Health Bull.* 210.
17. Clarke, B. G., and Moffet, C. E. (1941). *J. Ind. Hyg. Toxicol.* **23**, 176.
18. Flinn, R. H., *et al.* (1941). *U. S. Pub. Health Ser. Bull.* 270.
19. Jones, R. H. (1942). *J. Amer. Med. Ass.* **119**, 611.
20. Gordon, B., *et al.* (1949). *W. Va. Med. J.* **45**, 125.
21. Lainhart, W. S., *et al.* (1969). "Pneumoconiosis in Appalachian Bituminous Coal Miners." Govt. Print. Off., Washington, D. C.
22. Martin, J. E. (1953). *Amer. J. Pub. Health* **44**, 581.
23. Kerr, L. E. (1956). *Ind. Med. Surg.* **25**, 355.
24. Doyle, H. N., and Noehren, T. H. (1954). *U. S. Pub. Health Bibliogr. Ser.* 11.

25. Levine, M. D., and Hunter, M. B. (1957). *J. Amer. Med. Ass.* **163**, 1.
26. Lieben, J., Pendergrass, E., and McBride, W. W. (1961). *J. Occup. Med.* **3**, 493.
27. Baier, E. J., and Diakun, R. (1961). *J. Occup. Med.* **3**, 507.
28. Lieben, J., and Hill, P. C. (1962). *Pa. Med. J.* **65**, 1475.
29. McBride, W. W., Pendergrass, E., and Lieben, J. (1963). *J. Occup. Med.* **5**, 376.
30. Stoeckle, J. D., *et al.* (1961). *J. Chronic Dis.* **15**, 887.
31. U. S. Senate (1963). "Hearings on H. R. 10904." Labor, Health, Educ. Welfare Appropriations, 664.
32. Brown, M. C. (1965). *Mining Congr. J.* **51**, 44.
33. Lainhart, W. S., *et al.* (1968). *Arch. Environ. Health* **16**, 207.
34. Lieben, J. (1967). "Coal Miners' Pneumoconiosis in Pennsylvania—1967." *W. Va. School Med. Centen. Symp. Coal Workers' Pneumoconiosis.*
35. Davis, F. L., and Bowman, F. J. (1970). "Workmen's Compensation Law, State of West Virginia." W. Va. Workmen's Compens. Comm., Charleston, W. Va.
36. Enterline, P. E. (1964). *Amer. J. Pub. Health* **54**, 758.
37. Hyatt, R. E., Kisten, A. D., and Mahan, T. K. (1963). *Amer. Rev. Resp. Dis.* **89**, 387.
38. Gilson, J. C., *et al.* (1970). *Chest* **58**, 57.
39. International Labour Office (1970). "International Classification of Radiographs of Pneumoconioses." *Occup. Saf. Health Ser.* 22.
40. Pennsylvania Department of Health (1964). "Proceedings of the Governor's Conf. on Pneumoconiosis (Anthraco-silicosis)," Harrisburg, Pa.
41. Lee, D. H. K. (1971). *J. Occup. Med.* (in press).
42. International Conference on CWP. (1969). "Synopsis of the Work Session Proceedings." 10–12 Sept. Spindletop Res., Inc., Lexington, Ky.
43. Pendergrass, E. P. (1970). *Arch. Environ. Health* **20**, 545.
44. "Symposium on Respirable Coal Mine Dust Proceedings" (1970). Govt. Print. Off., Washington, D. C.
45. "National Conference on Medicine and the Federal Coal Mine Health and Safety Act of 1969" (1970). Washington, D. C.

2

Coal in the United States

Donald P. Schlick and Nicholas L. Fannick

Coal was first discovered in the United States in 1673 by Joliet and Marquette in Illinois. The first mining operations were begun in 1701 on the James River near Richmond, Va., but it was not until 1745 that bituminous coal was mined on a commercial basis.

The United States coal fields cover approximately 400,000 square miles or one-ninth of the total land area. Because of its utility and availability, coal has become a basic component of American industry—it generates more than half (51.8%) of the nations electricity; it is a necessary part of the vital iron and steel industries; and it is the basis of thousands of chemical by-products used by industrial and private consumers.

GEOLOGY AND CHEMISTRY

Geology

Most of the coal in the United States was formed during the Mississippian and Pennsylvanian geological epochs (Lower and Upper Carboniferous) about 250 million years ago. The coal found here is classed by four ranks: lignite, subbituminous, bituminous, and anthracite.

The fourth and lowest rank, lignite, is a soft, crumbly, brown-to-black coal that is somewhat more compact than peat. Lignite disintegrates rapidly in air and is liable to spontaneous combustion. It is mined on a limited basis.

Subbituminous coal, the third class, was formed under greater pressures than lignite. This caused additional loss of volatile constituents and

13

a corresponding increase in the relative content of fixed carbon. Although subbituminous coal is black and looks a great deal like bituminous, it weathers and slacks rapidly when exposed to air and is subject to spontaneous combustion if not properly stored.

Bituminous coal, second-class rank, is the most abundant and the most widely used for industrial power, railroad, and heating purposes. There is an almost endless list of slightly different grades of bituminous.

Anthracite, first-class rank, the highest grade of coal, has a brilliant luster and a hard, uniform texture. It was formed under greater pressure than bituminous—pressures resulting from the folding of the earth's surface into great mountain ranges. In the United States, anthracite is mined only in northeastern Pennsylvania.

The United States Geological Survey* estimated that as of 1 January 1967, the remaining coal reserve of the United States was 1,559,875 million short tons. The total reserves of the various ranks of coal are listed in Table I. See Fig. 1 for a map of coal areas in the United States.

TABLE I
TOTAL OF THE VARIOUS RANKS OF COAL

Rank of coal	Millions of short tons in reserve
Bituminous	671,049
Subbituminous	428,210
Lignite	447,647
Anthracite	12,969
Total, all ranks	1,559,875

Chemistry

United States coal is analyzed on the basis of four items: (i) water (moisture); (ii) mineral impurity (ash) left when the coal is completely burned; (iii) volatile matter, consisting of the gases driven out when the coal is heated; and (iv) fixed carbon, which represents the coke-like residue that burns at greater temperatures after the volatile matter is driven off.

Because there are so very many varieties of bituminous coal in the United States, a typical chemical analysis is not meaningful. Table II was extracted from a Bureau of Mines chart and lists analyses of different ranks of coal.

* Aueritt, Paul. Coal Resources of the United States, January 1, 1967. Bulletin 1275, Geological Survey, 1969.

TABLE II

ANALYSES OF DIFFERENT RANKS OF COAL[a]

Class by rank	State	County	Bed	Condition[b]	Proximate percent			Ultimate percent		
					Moisture	Volatile matter	Fixed carbon	Ash	Sulfur	Calor. value (B.T.U./lb)
1. Anthracite	Pa.	Lackawanna	Clark	1	4.3	5.1	81.0	9.6	0.8	12,880
2. High-volatile A bituminous coal	W. Va.	Marion	Pittsburgh	1	2.3	36.5	56.0	5.2	0.8	14,040
3. Subbituminous B coal	Wyo.	Sheridan	Monarch	1	22.2	33.2	40.3	4.3	0.5	9,610
4. Lignite	N.D.	McLean	(Unnamed)	1	36.8	27.8	29.5	5.9	0.9	7,000

[a] Source and analyses of coals selected to represent the various ranks of the Specifications for Classification of Coals by Rank adopted by the American Society for Testing and Materials. Prepared by W. A. Selvig, Bureau of Mines, U. S. Department of the Interior, Washington, D. C.

[b] Sample as received.

MINING METHODS

World production of coal totaled 3.08 billion tons in 1968. The United States supplied nearly 557 million tons of bituminous, anthracite, and lignite, or 18% of the world output in 1968.

Underground

Underground production of coal amounted to 344.1 million tons in 1968 or 63.1% of the United States production. Traditionally, underground coal is mined by the room-and-pillar mining system. In this mining method, main entries are driven into the coal seam and act as haulageways and aircourses. Side entries project into the seam from which coal is removed, forming "rooms."

Up to half of the coal is left in the form of pillars to support the roof.

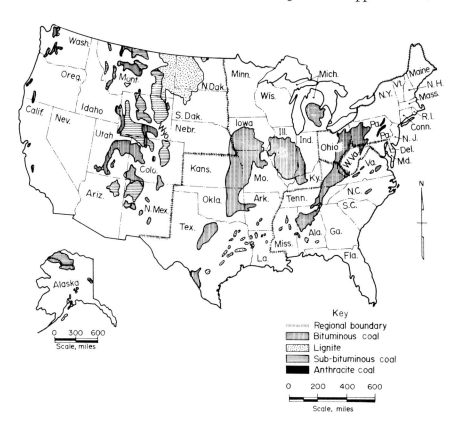

FIG. 1. Map of coal areas in the United States by class.

Conditions permitting, these pillars may be removed on retreat. Since the mid-1930's, coal mining has been mechanized to the point of almost eliminating the hand-loading system of yesteryear. Mechanical, or conventional, mining is characterized by separate machines for drilling, cutting, loading, and roof shoring. In recent years, continuous mining machines have been designed and developed which combine the cutting and loading. This advent of mechanization has revolutionized the mining industry and brought about a marked increase in productivity.

In longwall mining, the prevailing system in European coal mines, a planer or a plow extends along the entire work face (300–600 ft) and contains a coal conveyor. The plow or planer is pulled along the face and rips off coal.

This system has recently begun to gain acceptance in American mines. Coal tonnage mined in the United States by the longwall method increased threefold from 1966 to 1969, growing from 0.4% of all coal mined in 1966 to 1.2% in 1969. Even though these figures are small in an absolute sense, a trend of increasing use of longwall mining is apparent.

Strip Mining

Surface mining may be more economical than underground mining when the coal seam lies near the surface. In strip mining, the earth cover, or overburden, is removed by large power shovels. The exposed coal is then removed and loaded by smaller power shovels. Mining operations usually follow the coal seam until such time as the ratio of overburden to coal makes production uneconomical.

In 1968 production from surface mining amounted to 201.1 million tons, 33.9% of the total United States coal production. The fantastic growth of strip mining was made possible by the development of large-capacity equipment and new blasting agents. Strip mining has the advantages over underground mining of a greater output per man and a resulting lower cost per ton.

Augering

Auger mining, only recently developed, is gaining rapid acceptance. In 1968, it produced 15.3 million tons, or 3% of the total United States production.

When strip mines encounter an overburden too thick for economical removal, they sometimes revert to augering. These strip mines leave seams of coal exposed along what is commonly called a highwall. Large augers bore horizontal holes from the highwall into the seam, much as a carpenter's auger bores holes into wood. The coal is removed from inside the seam through a tube and screw.

The depth to which augering is carried out depends to a large extent on the coal thickness, whether the seams roll or are flat, and if they are strong enough to stand after penetration and not foul the auger.

Punch mining is similar to auger mining in that it is considered a secondary system of mining of coal that normally would be lost owing to the uneconomical overburden ratio. Punch mining employs conventional or continuous mining equipment and underground mining methods to win the coal from the highwall left by the stripping operation.

RESPIRABLE DUST SAMPLING EQUIPMENT

In the United States, respirable dust is measured on a mass concentration basis by two types of respirable size gravimetric samplers: the personal sampler and the MRE instrument. These two-stage instruments continuously sample air from the worker's breathing zone during the full working shift. The atmosphere is drawn through the devices by portable battery-operated pumps powered by nickel–cadmium batteries. Both instruments are battery operated, portable, and instrinsically safe for use in United States coal mines.

The coal mine dust personal sampler was developed by the United States Bureau of Mines. The first stage, a 10-mm nylon cyclone, performs as an elutriator or size selector. Penetration conforms to a curve which is in close agreement with the criterion for dust deposition in the lungs reported by the United States Atomic Energy Commission. The second stage is a membrane filter that collects the respirable fraction of the dust. The dust collected is weighed to the nearest 0.1 mg, and concentrations are expressed in milligrams per cubic meter of air sampled.

The second instrument used to collect respirable dust samples is an instrument developed at the Mining Research Establishment of the National Coal Board at Isleworth, Great Britain. Air is drawn at the rate of 2.5 liters/minute through a four-plate horizontal elutriator, and the penetrating respirable fraction of the dust is collected on a 55-mm-diameter polyvinyl chloride membrane filter. Penetration characteristics of the elutriator (see Fig. 2) agree with the size criteria specified at the Johannesburg Conference. Mass concentrations of samples collected by the MRE instruments are evaluated by weighing the dust retained on the filter to the nearest 0.1 mg. The dust concentration is reported as milligrams of respirable dust per cubic meter of air sampled.

Each instrument has its advantages and disadvantages. The horizontal

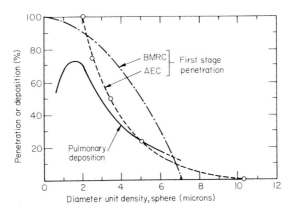

FIG. 2. Specifications for size selective performance.

elutriator-type sampler is bulky, cannot be attached to a miner to determine his dust exposure during the working shift, and is relatively sensi-
tive to horizontal positioning. Its advantages are the consistencies of an
empirical relationship between results obtained with this instrument and
those obtained with the midget impinger collected under specified
conditions.

The advantages of the personal cyclone sampler for gravimetric determination of respirable dust are: the device is light in weight and is portable; positioning of the sampler does not materially affect its operation;
and the coarse fraction can be readily recovered for analysis. The disadvantages are that the design characteristics cannot be precalculated,
the rate of airflow through the cyclone affects the collection efficiency,
particle penetration through the cyclone is reported to decrease with
concentration, and agglomeration and disaggregation can occur within
the cyclone, causing the characteristics of the collected sample to differ
from those of the dust cloud.

The penetration curve of the cyclone's respirable size fraction differs
from that of the MRE instrument. However, the ratio of the concentrations collected in sampling under controlled test conditions and in actual
coal mine tests appears to be nearly constant.

In addition to the previously mentioned gravimetric respirable dust
samplers, which are required to fulfill sampling requirements under the
Federal Coal Mine Health and Safety Act of 1969, the impinger-type
instrument is used in coal mines for engineering investigations.

Although impingers are not used extensively outside this country, they
have been in use in the United States since 1922 to collect samples for
the determination of dust exposures. Most of the information correlating

degree of dustiness with physiological effects has been obtained by use of the impinger and standardized light-field count methods.

The Greenburg–Smith impinger was developed at the Bureau of Mines in cooperation with the U. S. Public Health Service in 1922. The midget impinger was designed in 1937 to overcome the objections to the use of the early impinger, which was bulky and heavy and had a high power dissipation rate. The newer device is a small-scale duplicate of the standard instrument in every respect except that it operates at an impinging velocity of 70 instead of 100 m/second and samples at a rate of 0.1 instead of 1 ft³/minute. The development of the midget impinger greatly extended the practical convenience and usefulness of this method of dust sampling, because it provided the investigator with a light, small, hand-operated device for use in underground coal mines. Presently, intrinsically safe, battery-powered sampling pumps are available for operating midget impinger samplers.

MINE ENVIRONMENT

Dust Concentrations in Large Underground Coal Mines

In April 1968 the Bureau of Mines initiated a study of dust exposures in selected large underground bituminous coal mines. The objective of this comprehensive study was to obtain data on the respirable dust exposures of coal miners. These data would then be used for correlation with medical data obtained by the U. S. Public Health Service on the same coal miners. It was hoped that this study would provide information which would be useful in the development of a respirable dust standard and the determination of the effects of dust on the progression of pneumoconiosis.

The study was limited to mines that employed more than 20 men and had a producing life in excess of 10 years. All major bituminous coal fields were assessed. The study included a variety of production methods and mining systems, resulting in an overview of mining conditions indicative of those found in the bituminous-coal mining industry. During the study, no attempt was made to alter mining methods which would result in changing worker's dust exposures.

Nearly 2000 samples were evaluated to determine occupational respirable dust exposures in underground coal mines. Table III illustrates the mean dust concentrations found in the 29 mines that were studied.

The respirable dust exposures listed in Table III are indicative of concentrations found throughout the bituminous-coal mining industry at the time of this survey. It should be noted that these exposures are neither

TABLE III

MINE MEAN DUST CONCENTRATIONS BY OCCUPATION[a]

Occupation	No. of mines	No. of samples	Dust concentration (mg/m³)				Low, high and mean concentration (mg/m³)			
			<1.6	1.61–2.4	2.41–2.9	>2.9	Low	High	Mean	MRE equivalent
Continuous miner operator	21	178	2	2	4	13	0.02	21.44	4.08	7.7
Continuous miner helper	19	131	4	3	2	10	0.44	18.90	3.47	6.5
Cutting machine operator	15	98	1	6	2	6	0.71	15.42	3.69	6.9
Cutting machine helper	8	37	1	3	—	4	0.77	14.70	4.45	8.4
Coal drill operator	9	59	3	—	1	5	0.42	12.94	3.55	6.7
Loading machine operator	18	97	2	1	2	13	0.25	39.56	3.75	7.1
Loading machine helper	6	31	—	3	—	3	0.50	14.48	3.17	6.0
Roof bolter operator	25	296	6	9	6	4	0.09	38.50	2.46	4.6
Shuttle car operator	27	463	17	7	3	—	0.12	10.50	1.45	2.7
Beltman	7	32	2	3	1	1	0.42	4.97	1.85	3.5
Boomboy	6	20	5	—	—	1	0.23	5.88	1.30	2.4
Timberman	12	49	7	1	—	4	0.38	11.74	2.49	4.7
Shotfirer	12	83	5	2	2	3	0.62	56.97	3.15	5.9
Supplyman	8	24	5	1	1	1	0.05	9.36	1.59	3.0
Mechanic	19	142	17	2	—	—	0.06	5.43	1.10	2.1
Section Foreman	28	236	19	4	2	3	0.14	14.51	1.69	3.2
Percent of Total	—	—	40	19	11	30	—	—	—	—

[a] Sample taken with the personal sampler.

presumed nor implied to be representative of dust concentrations in the mines prior to this survey.

An analysis of the data indicates that (i) a significant number of occupations has respirable dust exposures in excess of the proposed legislative limits, (ii) the lightest dust exposures were recorded on the cutting machine helper, (iii) water and face ventilation were the only measures used to control airborne dust, and (iv) ventilating air entering working places in some cases contained a considerable amount of dust.

The respirable dust standard in the Federal Coal Mine Health and Safety Act of 1969 is for dust containing less than 5% SiO_2 (quartz). Table IV shows results of analysis from quartz from samples taken during

TABLE IV
Quartz Percentage in Mine Atmospheres

Mine	Quartz (SiO_2)	
	Respirable	Gross
A-1	1.6	—
A-2	1.3	1.4
A-3	.9	1.2
A-4	.4	.4
A-5	1.1	.6
A-6	1.5	1.0
A-7	1.0	2.3
A-8	—	—
A-9	—	—
B-1	1.1	.8
B-2	.8	—
B-3	2.9	2.1
B-4	2.4	2.1
B-5	.9	1.1
B-6	—	—
B-7	—	—
C-1	2.2	1.7
C-2	1.8	1.2
C-3	3.1	2.4
C-4	1.3	.9
C-5	2.3	1.5
C-6	2.2	1.5
C-7	—	—
C-8	—	—
D-1	2.0	1.9
D-2	—	—
D-3	—	—
D-4	—	—
E-1	1.0	.5

this study. In all mines studied, the quartz content was below 5%, with an average of 1.5%.

Dust Concentrations in Small Underground Coal Mines

In September 1969 the Bureau of Mines conducted a study to determine respirable dust exposures in 12 small bituminous coal mines. The objective of this study was similar to that of the study conducted in large mines. The criteria for selection of mines were employment under six men and production of less than 100 tons/shift.

An analysis of this study produced the following conclusions:

1. Slightly over 50% of the miners monitored were subjected to exposures of less than 3.0 mg/m³, and nearly 80% were subjected to exposures of less than 4.5 mg/m³. All measurements were taken with personal samplers and were converted to MRE equivalents.

2. In most cases, excessive respirable dust concentrations resulted from lack of face ventilation.

3. All investigators reported that respirable dust levels could be markedly reduced by employing face ventilation techniques.

4. Higher dust concentrations were recorded on miners working at distances well beyond their source of fresh ventilating air.

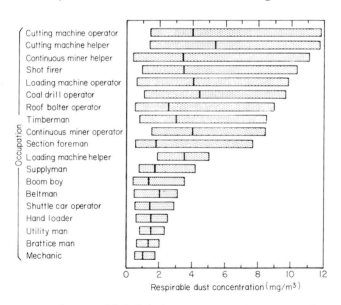

FIG. 3. Mean and range of full shift dust exposures relative to specific occupations in bituminous coal mines.

5. The graph in Fig. 3 shows dust exposures relative to specific occupations, measured with the personal sampler. The graph in Fig. 4 is a comparison of the dust exposures (converted to MRE values) from large and small mines.

Dust Concentrations in Aboveground Mining Facilities

In the summer of 1970, the Bureau of Mines conducted a study to determine respirable dust exposures in 39 strip mines, auger mines, and preparation plants. The facilities chosen were representative of the industry in size and methods of operation.

An analysis of this study produced the following conclusions:

1. Eighty-eight percent of all workers had exposures of less than 2 mg/m^3. All measurements were taken with personal samplers and were converted to MRE equivalents.

2. In most cases, excessive respirable dust concentrations were found

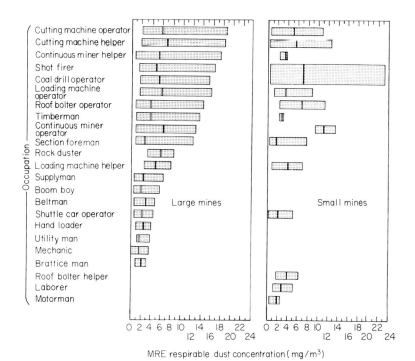

FIG. 4. Range and average respirable dust concentration for specific occupations (MRE).

among the laborer or repairman occupations where the excessive exposure resulted from exposure while in a confining area.

3. Exposures at strip and auger mines are presumably less in winter months when vehicle windows are closed.

Table V indicates that the mean and median exposures at aboveground facilities were much less than the exposures underground.

TABLE V

SUMMARY OF THIRTY-NINE SURFACE STUDIES

Type of facility	No. of samples	% < 1 mg/m³	% < 2 mg/m³	% < 3 mg/m³	Mean	Median
Auger	50	68	86	90	1.1	0.7
Preparation plant	516	57	84	93	1.3	0.9
Strip	416	79	93	97	0.8	0.6
	982	67	88	94	1.1	0.7

Control of Respirable Dust

In general, control measures used which reduce respirable dust are limited to water and ventilation. Water infused into the coal seam has produced limited results. In 1957 the Bureau of Mines reported that water infusion did not materially reduce respirable dust. Some reduction was later reported in continuous mining, but the reduction was insufficient to meet legislated requirements.

Water sprays are employed extensively throughout the coal mining industry to abate concentrations of total airborne dust, as well as respirable dust. Spraying systems are used on the coal mining machines as well as at loading points and coal transfer points. To reduce respirable dust, water sprays must produce a very fine mist to be effective on particles 1 micron or less in size. Producing the necessary quantity of small droplets of water in the form of a mist which is required to allay respirable dust has not been completely successful.

After data from previous studies were initially assessed, it became increasingly apparent that the single most important parameter affecting the abatement of respirable dust was ventilation. In an effort to further refine the effect of ventilation, the Bureau launched a short-term technical study in mines on the control of respirable coal mine dust by ventilation. Results of these tests clearly indicated that under certain conditions, face-generated dust could be effectively confined, captured, and conducted to return airways. Figure 5 illustrates test results of face-generated concen-

D. P. Schlick and N. L. Fannick

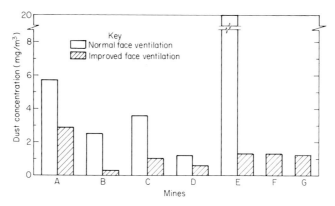

FIG. 5. Face-generated respirable dust concentration at continuous mining machine.

trations of respirable dust at continuous mining machines recorded during this study. Thus, in some situations the technology exists which can greatly reduce harmful concentrations of respirable dust. However, adapting this technology to existing mining equipment and underground conditions will, in some cases, prove difficult. For instance, in coal seams where the total mining height is less than 48 in., it is difficult to provide the space required to make this technology applicable. Also in retreat or pillar mining, there may be a problem in maintaining the velocity of air required to establish control. Finally, and as a direct result of this study, it was determined that the amount of respirable dust entering the section may contribute to high dust concentrations.

PART 2
CLINICAL CHARACTERISTICS

3

Extent and Distribution of Respiratory Effects

William S. Lainhart and W. Keith C. Morgan

While several studies have been carried out in the United States on the prevalence of coal workers' pneumoconiosis, almost no attempt has been made to relate environmental conditions in the mines to the prevalence of the disease as detected radiographically. The Federal Coal Mine Health and Safety Act of 1969 and the studies now being conducted by the U. S. Public Health Service should do much to overcome this deficiency.

Reliable data concerning the frequency of various respiratory diseases as they occur in the coal mining population are scanty; nonetheless, it is fairly well accepted that coal miners have a higher prevalence of lung disease than does the general male population (1–3). The cause of this increased respiratory morbidity and mortality is not completely understood and, moreover, cannot be attributed to a single respiratory disease or any particular set of circumstances that the coal miner encounters in the performance of his job. Several respiratory diseases occur more frequently in miners. In some instances, e.g., CWP, there is a direct relationship between the inhalation of coal dust and the disease that results. However, most of the increased respiratory morbidity and mortality appears to be a consequence of nonspecific obstructive airway disease. Furthermore, although there is little doubt that obstructive airway disease occurs more frequently in coal miners, there is at present no conclusive evidence that coal dust inhalation is concerned in its etiology (4).

Prevalence Studies in the United States

From 1963 to 1965, 3602 working bituminous-coal miners (from mines with more than 15 miners employed underground) had a radiologic examination of their chest. The miners worked in mines in the three major geographic regions of coal production in the United States: Appalachia (55 mines located in 20 counties), southern Illinois and Indiana (12 mines located in eight counties), and Utah (five mines located in a single county) (Table I) (5).

TABLE I

WORKING UNITED STATES COAL MINERS (5) EXAMINED IN 1963–1965

Number, age and underground experience	Appalachia	Illinois–Indiana	Utah	Total
No. contacted	2751	520	591	3862
No. examined and %	2549 (92.7%)	477 (91.7%)	576 (97.5%)	3602 (93.3%)
No. not examined	202	43	15	260
Average age (yr)	46.5	47.7	50.5	—
Standard deviation (yr)	9.7	11.4	8.6	—
Average underground (yr)	21.6	20.0	19.6	—
Standard deviation (yr)	11.0	11.4	13.1	—

The controlled probability sampling method outlined elsewhere (6) was used to study the population. Approximately 4% of the working miners in Appalachia and 10% in the Illinois–Indiana and Utah coal fields were asked to participate. The response varied from 91.7% in the Illinois–Indiana area to 97.5% in the Utah area with an overall participation of 93.3%. The miners in Utah were slightly older and had slightly fewer average years underground than their counterparts in Illinois–Indiana or Appalachia, although this difference was not statistically significant (Table I). Aside from the radiologic examination, participants answered a questionnaire concerning chest illnesses, smoking, and respiratory symptoms. An occupational history was taken and some simple tests of pulmonary function were performed. Further reference to this part of the study is made later.

The principal occupation of each working coal miner was considered to be that to which he had devoted the most number of years during his work in the coal mines. Almost one-half of the Appalachian miners (42.0%), compared to about 36% of the other two groups of miners, had worked mainly at the face (Table II). The distribution of workers in the other mining jobs was similar in the various geographic regions, although there were more surface workers in the Utah region than in the Illinois–Indiana.

TABLE II

PRINCIPAL OCCUPATION OF WORKING COAL MINERS (5)

Principal occupation	Appalachia		Illinois–Indiana		Utah	
	No.	%	No.	%	No.	%
Underground						
Face	1068	42.0	173	36.3	208	36.3
Transportation	548	21.5	95	19.9	101	17.6
Maintenance	360	14.2	102	21.4	84	14.7
Miscellaneous	174	6.8	21	4.4	44	7.7
	2150	84.5	391	82.0	437	76.3
Surface						
Transportation	47	1.8	11	2.3	9	1.6
Maintenance	107	4.2	41	8.6	50	8.7
Tipple	162	6.4	20	4.2	52	9.1
Strip mining	67	2.6	0	—	0	—
Miscellaneous	12	0.5	14	2.9	25	4.3
	395	15.5	86	18.0	136	23.7
Underground + surface	2545		477		573	
Unknown	4		0		3	

A standard posteroanterior chest radiograph (14 in. $\times$ 17 in.) was taken of 3579 of the 3602 coal miners examined. The films were taken at 72 in. with the use of 200-mA mobile unit equipment with a phototimer. Exposed films were developed in the unit, usually at the mine site, and immediately screened by the team physician. In the event of a radiograph's being considered to be technically unsatisfactory, the miner was contacted and requested to return for a repeat examination. All films were then sent to the Occupational Health Research and Training Facility, Cincinnati, Ohio, for recording and distribution to a panel of radiologists. Each radiograph was read independently by the panel members using the U. S. Public Health Service modification of the International Labour Organization Radiological Classification of Chest Films (Fig. 1) (7).

A radiograph was classified as negative for pneumoconiosis when there was no radiographic evidence of this disease in the lung fields. Suspected pneumoconiosis (classification "Z") included the following possibilities:

(a) An area of nodulation suggestive of pneumoconiosis but not of sufficient extent to be included in Category 1 (i.e., not an area ". . . equivalent to at least the second and third anterior rib spaces of either side")

TYPE OF OPACITY	FILM QUALITY		NO PNEUMO-CONIOSIS	SUSPECT	PNEUMOCONIOSIS					
					SMALL OPACITIES			LARGE OPACITIES*		
QUANTITATIVE FEATURES	UNSAT FILM	POOR FILM	O	Z	1	2	3	A	B	C
QUALITATIVE FEATURES					p q r	p q r	p q r			
ADDITIONAL SYMBOLS	ax ca cn co cv di em es hi pl px rl tb tba nt np									
FILM QUALITY	UNSATISFACTORY FILM — IMPOSSIBLE TO READ POOR FILM - DETAILED CLASSIFICATION DIFFICULT									
NO PNEUMO-CONIOSIS	O - NO RADIOGRAPHIC EVIDENCE OF PNEUMOCONIOSIS IN LUNG FIELDS.									
SUSPECT OPACITIES	Z - SHADOWS WHICH MAY BE PNEUMOCONIOTIC BUT WHICH ARE INSUFFICIENT FOR THE FILM TO BE PLACED IN ONE OF THE CATEGORIES CLASSIFYING THE SMALL OPACITIES.									

PNEUMOCONIOSIS

SMALL OPACITIES	THE CATEGORIZATION DEPENDS ON THE EXTENT AND PROFUSION OF THE OPACITIES : 1 A NUMBER OF OPACITIES IN AN AREA EQUIVALENT TO AT LEAST THE SECOND AND THIRD ANTERIOR RIB SPACES OF EITHER SIDE, AND AT THE MOST, NOT GREATER THAN ONE THIRD OF THE TWO LUNG FIELDS COMBINED. 2 OPACITIES MORE DIFFUSE THAN IN CATEGORY 1 WHICH MAY BE DISTRIBUTED OVER THE WHOLE OR NEARLY THE WHOLE OF THE LUNG FIELDS 3 VERY NUMEROUS OPACITIES DISTRIBUTED OVER THE WHOLE, OR NEARLY THE WHOLE OF THE LUNG FIELDS	THESE ARE CLASSIFIED ACCORDING TO THE GREATEST DIAMETER OF THE PREDOMINANT OPACITIES AND DENOTED BY THE FOLLOWING SYMBOLS : p - GREATEST DIAMETER UP TO AND INCLUDING 1.5 mm q - GREATEST DIAMETER FROM 1.5 mm UP TO AND INCLUDING 3 mm r - GREATEST DIAMETER FROM 3 mm UP TO AND INCLUDING 1 cm
LARGE OPACITIES	A - AN OPACITY HAVING A GREATEST DIAMETER EXCEEDING 1 cm AND UP TO AND INCLUDING 5 cm OR SEVERAL OPACITIES EACH GREATER THAN 1 cm, THE SUM OF WHOSE GREATEST DIAMETERS DOES NOT EXCEED 5 cm B - ONE OR MORE OPACITIES LARGER OR MORE NUMEROUS THAN THOSE IN CATEGORY A WHOSE COMBINED AREA DOES NOT EXCEED ONE THIRD OF THE VISIBLE RIGHT LUNG C - ONE OR MORE OPACITIES WHOSE COMBINED AREA EXCEEDS ONE THIRD OF THE VISIBLE RIGHT LUNG FIELD.	
EGGSHELL CALCIFICATIONS (ES)	SPECIFIC CRITERIA FOR IDENTIFYING EGGSHELL CALCIFICATIONS AS EVIDENCE OF SILICOSIS: (1) THE PRESENCE OF SHELL-LIKE CALCIFICATIONS MEASURING UP TO 2 mm IN THICKNESS IN THE PERIPHERAL ZONE OF AT LEAST TWO LYMPH NODES (2) THESE CALCIFICATIONS MAY BE SOLID OR BROKEN (3) IN AT LEAST ONE OF THE LYMPH NODES THE RING-LIKE SHADOW MUST BE COMPLETE. (4) THE CENTRAL PORTION OF THE LYMPH NODE MAY SHOW, IN ADDITION, SPECKLED CALCIFICATION. (5) THE AFFECTED LYMPH NODE MUST BE AT LEAST 1 cm IN ITS GREATEST DIAMETER.	

CODE FOR ADDITIONAL SYMBOLS

ax - SUSPECT COALESCENCE OF SMALL PNEUMOCONIOTIC OPACITIES
ca - SUSPECT CANCER OF THE LUNG
cn - CALCIFICATION IN SMALL OPACITIES
co - ABNORMALITIES OF THE CARDIAC OUTLINE. TO BE REPLACED BY "cp-cor pulmonale" IF THIS CONDITION IS STRONGLY SUSPECTED
cv - CAVITY
di - SIGNIFICANT DISPLACEMENT OR DISTORTION OF THE INTRATHORACIC ORGANS
em - EMPHYSEMA

es - EGGSHELL CALCIFICATION OF LYMPH NODES
hi - APPRECIABLE ENLARGEMENT OF THE HILAR SHADOWS
pl - ABNORMALITY OF THE PLEURA
px - PNEUMOTHORAX
rl - PNEUMOCONIOSIS MODIFIED BY THE RHEUMATOID PROCESS
tb - OPACITIES SUGGESTIVE OF INACTIVE TUBERCULOSIS, EXCLUDING THE CALCIFIED PRIMARY COMPLEX.
tba - OPACITIES SUGGESTIVE OF ACTIVE TUBERCULOSIS
nt - NONTUBERCULOUS INFECTION
np - PROBABLY NOT PNEUMOCONIOSIS

* THE BACKGROUND OF SMALL OPACITIES SHOULD BE SPECIFIED AS FAR AS POSSIBLE.

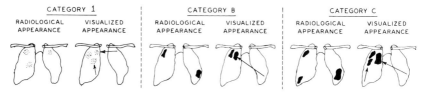

CATEGORY 1		CATEGORY B		CATEGORY C	
RADIOLOGICAL APPEARANCE	VISUALIZED APPEARANCE	RADIOLOGICAL APPEARANCE	VISUALIZED APPEARANCE	RADIOLOGICAL APPEARANCE	VISUALIZED APPEARANCE

FIG. 1. International radiological classification of chest films modified for U. S. Public Health Service chest studies.

(b) An area of suspected nodulation that might be confused with normal lung markings

(c) A film showing a large opacity (of A, B, or C size) consistent with pneumoconiosis but having a background that either could not be defined or did not show definite nodulation

(d) A film showing an infiltrative lesion that could be due to tuberculosis, cancer, or some other condition, but that aroused the suspicion of the reader as to the pneumoconiotic etiology of the lesion.

Simple pneumoconiosis included only small opacities (up to and including 1 cm in diameter) in the area of the lung equivalent to, or greater than, the second and third anterior rib interspaces of either side of the chest. A radiograph was classified as showing complicated pneumoconiosis when there were one or more large opacities (greater than 1 cm in diameter) regardless of the background of small opacities. A roentgenogram with a classification of either simple or complicated pneumoconiosis was considered "definite" pneumoconiosis, as opposed to one classified as "suspect" pneumoconiosis. The panel held periodic conferences to discuss cases in which disagreements in readings had occurred. After discussion, concensus readings were assigned to each case on the basis of the discussion of the three original readings.

Radiological Findings

The percentage of working miners showing definite radiological evidence of pneumoconiosis (i.e., simple and complicated) varied from approximately 10% in Appalachia through 6% in Illinois–Indiana to approximately 4% in Utah (Table III).

TABLE III

PNEUMOCONIOSIS IN WORKING COAL MINERS (5) BY
ROENTGENOGRAPHIC CATEGORY

Pneumoconiosis roentgenographic (category)	Appalachia		Illinois–Indiana		Utah	
	No.	%	No.	%	No.	%
None	2146	84.9	372	78.5	543	94.3
Suspect	135	5.3	73	15.4	11	1.9
Simple	172	6.8	22	4.6	18	3.1
Complicated	76	3.0	7	1.5	4	0.7
	2529		474		576	
No roentgenograms	20		3		0	

Definite pneumoconiosis (either simple or complicated) was seen primarily in underground workers (Fig. 2 and Table IV). The same relation between the three geographic areas held, i.e., 11% pneumoconiosis in underground Appalachian miners, 7.5% in Illinois–Indiana miners, and almost 5% in Utah miners.

Within the broad occupational groups, as shown in Fig. 3 and Table V,

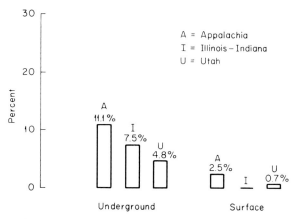

FIG. 2. Distribution of definite pneumoconiosis among working coal miners by comparison of pneumoconiosis in underground and surface workers.

there was more roentgenographic evidence of pneumoconiosis among face workers than among transportation, maintenance, or miscellaneous workers in Illinois–Indiana. In this context, it is pertinent to point out that the large percentage of subjects with pneumoconiosis among miscellaneous workers in the Illinois–Indiana area was based on the data from only 21 workers.

In Appalachia, cutting and loading machine operators (at the coal

TABLE IV

DEFINITE PNEUMOCONIOSIS AMONG WORKING COAL MINERS (5)

Pneumoconiosis among working groups	Appalachia		Illinois–Indiana		Utah	
	No.	%	No.	%	No.	%
Underground workers						
With pneumoconiosis	237	11.1	29	7.5	21	4.8
Without pneumoconiosis	1895	—	360	—	416	—
	2132		389		437	
Surface workers						
With pneumoconiosis	10	2.5	0	0.0	1	0.7
Without pneumoconiosis	383	—	85	—	136	—
	393		85		137	
Total with roentgenograms	2525		474		573	
Unknown history or no roentgenograms	24		3		3	
	2549		477		576	

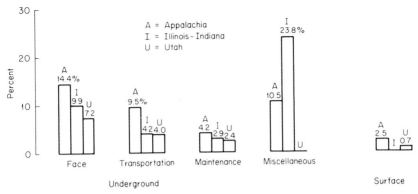

FIG. 3. Distribution of definite pneumoconiosis among working coal miners in relation to work location.

face) showed radiologic evidence of pneumoconiosis twice as frequently as did the other face workers. In all geographic areas, motormen and brakemen showed such evidence about four times as often as other transportation workers, although still much less frequently than the cutting and loading machine operators (Fig. 4, Table VI).

Radiologic evidence of definite pneumoconiosis varies with both age and years underground (Fig. 5). The effect of years underground appears to outweigh the effect of age. There was little radiological change with less than 10 years underground, even in the older age group where one might assume more mining experience on the basis of age alone. The marked change occurred after 20 years of underground mining, especially in Appalachia where more miners were examined than in the other two geographic areas.

Relationship of Prevalence to Rank of Coal Mined

In 1942 Hart and Aslett put forward the hypothesis that there is a relationship between the rank of coal mined and the prevalence of coal workers' pneumoconiosis (8). Studies in both Britain and the United States have yielded support for this theory (9). The term "rank" refers to certain properties and characteristics of coal that are described in the American Society for Testing and Materials (10). The range extends from anthracite at one extreme to lignite at the other. The higher ranked coals are in general the oldest, contain the most fixed carbon, have the greatest calorific value, and contain the least volatile matter.

The studies described above make it apparent that there is a wide variation in prevalence of CWP in the three regions surveyed by the Public Health Service. Although there are differences between the time

TABLE V

DEFINITE PNEUMOCONIOSIS AMONG WORKING COAL MINERS,
UNDERGROUND WORKERS, AND SURFACE WORKERS (5)

Pneumoconiosis among working groups	Appalachia		Illinois– Indiana		Utah	
	No.	%	No.	%	No.	%
Underground workers						
Face workers						
With pneumoconiosis	152	14.4	17	9.9	15	7.2
Without pneumoconiosis	906	—	154	—	193	—
	1058		171		208	
Transportation workers						
With pneumoconiosis	52	9.5	4	4.2	4	4.0
Without pneumoconiosis	493	—	91	—	97	—
	545		95		101	
Maintenance workers						
With pneumoconiosis	15	4.2	3	2.9	2	2.4
Without pneumoconiosis	342	—	99	—	82	—
	357		102		84	
Miscellaneous workers						
With pneumoconiosis	18	10.5	5	23.8	0	0.0
Without pneumoconiosis	154	—	16	—	44	—
	172		21		44	
Surface workers						
With pneumoconiosis	10	2.5	0	0.0	1	0.7
Without pneumoconiosis	383	—	85	—	135	—
	393		85		136	
Total with roentgenograms	2525		474		573	
Unknown history or no roentgenograms	24		3		3	
	2549		477		576	

spent underground in the three regions, these are relatively small and alone cannot account for the variation in prevalence. In contrast to the mines studied in Illinois–Indiana and Utah, which are confined to a few counties, the Appalachian mines ranged over a wide area and several states (Kentucky, Pennsylvania, Alabama, Virginia, and West Virginia). The number of miners examined at the different mines was statistically too small and there were too many other variables to allow comparison of prevalence rates between different areas of Appalachia except in one instance that is referred to later. Nonetheless, it is possible to make some correlation between the rank of coal mined and the prevalence rates in the three regions, if Appalachia is regarded as one area.

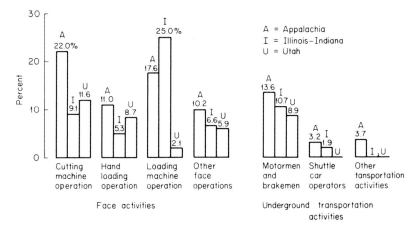

FIG. 4. Distribution of definite pneumoconiosis among working coal workers by type of operation.

The coal from the mines included in the study in Illinois and Indiana is low ranked and has a fixed carbon content of around 48–54%. This is the same order as is found in the Pittsburgh seam. The mines in Carbon County, Utah, contain even more volatile coal with a somewhat lower rank. Turning to Appalachia, the rank varies markedly from region to region. The highest ranked coal is found in the anthracite mines of eastern Pennsylvania; however, this region was not included in the study. The coal mined in central Pennsylvania is of medium rank, while in western Pennsylvania where the Pittsburgh seam predominates, the coal is of low rank. Similarly in northern West Virginia, the coal is volatile and of low rank, while in Wyoming, McDowell, and the other regions of the southern part of the state, the coal is less volatile and of higher rank.

As already stated, with one exception that is dealt with later, it is not possible to compare prevalence and rank in different areas of Appalachia from the U. S. Public Health Service survey. However, several other studies have been carried out which allow an attempt to be made to relate these factors. Thus Lieben and his colleagues carried out studies in eastern, central, and western Pennsylvania (11–13). Participation was voluntary and varied to a great extent. Moreover, other variables were present, e.g., years spent underground. Nonetheless, there was a definite transition from east to west in the percentage of working miners with radiological evidence of definite pneumoconiosis, viz. 18% in eastern Pennsylvania, 21% in central Pennsylvania,* and 9% in western Pennsylvania.

* The figures for central Pennsylvania are probably inaccurate since participation was poor.

TABLE VI

DEFINITE PNEUMOCONIOSIS BY SPECIFIC UNDERGROUND FACE
AND TRANSPORTATION ACTIVITIES (5)

Pneumoconiosis among working miners	Appalachia		Illinois–Indiana		Utah	
	No.	%	No.	%	No.	%
Face activities						
Cutting machine operators						
With pneumoconiosis	51	22.0	3	9.1	8	11.6
Without pneumoconiosis	181	—	30	—	61	—
	232		33		69	
Hand loaders						
With pneumoconiosis	44	11.0	1	5.3	2	8.7
Without pneumoconiosis	355	—	18	—	21	—
	399		19		23	
Loading machine operators						
With pneumoconiosis	32	17.6	7	25.0	1	2.1
Without pneumoconiosis	150	—	21	—	47	—
	182		28		48	
Other face activities						
With pneumoconiosis	25	10.2	6	6.6	4	5.9
Without pneumoconiosis	220	—	85	—	64	—
	245		91		68	
Underground transportation activities						
Motormen and brakemen						
With pneumoconiosis	45	13.6	3	10.7	4	8.9
Without pneumoconiosis	287	—	25	—	41	—
	332		28		45	
Shuttle car operators						
With pneumoconiosis	5	3.2	1	1.9	0	0.0
Without pneumoconiosis	153	—	51	—	38	—
	158		52		38	
Other transportation activities						
With pneumoconiosis	2	3.7	0	0.0	0	0.0
Without pneumoconiosis	52	—	15	—	18	—
	54		15		18	
Total with roentgenograms	1603		266		309	
Unknown history or no roentgenograms	13		2		0	
	1616		268		309	

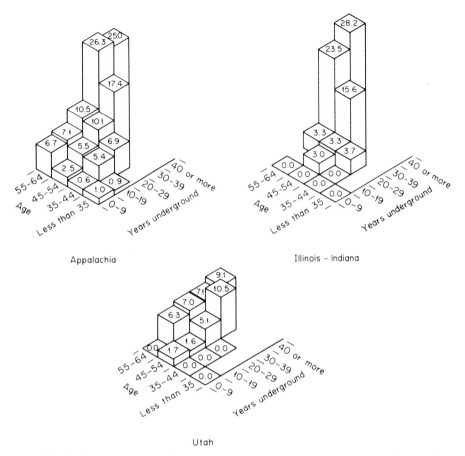

Appalachia   Illinois – Indiana

Utah

FIG. 5. Distribution of definite pneumoconiosis by age and years underground.

Several community studies which included miners have also been carried out in West Virginia in areas having coal of different ranks. That of Higgins took place in Marion County (14), whereas the U. S. Public Health Service, as part of the larger prevalence study, selected two communities in West Virginia—Richwood, and Mullens—for comparison (15). These towns originally were selected because they allowed comparison of two nonmining populations with comparable populations of coal miners in geographically distinct areas of the state. In this study there was a slight difference in the duration of working history, the mean time spent in coal mining being 19.2 years in Richwood compared with 22.3 years in Mullens. This, however, is not sufficient to account for the markedly greater prevalence among miners in Mullens. (See pp. 52–56.)

TABLE VII

Regional Prevalence of Coal Workers' Pneumoconiosis in Appalachia, Coal Seams Which Occur in Each Region, and the Rank of Coal Present in the Seams

Region and study	Characteristics of study group	Mean age (yr)	Mean age of miners with coal workers' pneumoconiosis (yr)	Percentage participation	Total examined roentgenographically	Number with coal workers' pneumoconiosis[a]	Number with progressive massive fibrosis	Percentage with coal workers' pneumoconiosis who had progressive massive fibrosis	Rank of coal mined	Coal seams
Eastern Pennsylvania, McBride et al. (12)	Working miners, 20 yr and more	48.5	55	Approx. 60	1300	235 (18)	182	77	High rank, anthracite	—
Central Pennsylvania, Lieben et al. (13)	Working miners, 20 yr and more	46.5	50.5	25	4176	885 (21)	497	51	Almost entirely of medium or high rank; low volatility	Upper and lower Freeport; upper, middle, and lower Kittanning; Brookville, Sewickley, Clarion, Redstone

Western Pennsylvania, McBride et al. (14)	Working miners, 20 yr and more	47	52	68	8237	681 (9)	345	51	Almost entirely of low rank; high volatility	Pittsburgh, Waynesburg, Sewickley, Redstone, upper Freeport
Northern West Virginia, Marion Co., Higgins (15)	Working miners, 20 yr and more	48	52.5	More than 80	306	21 (7)	0	0	Mainly medium or low rank; high volatility	Pittsburgh
Southern West Virginia, Mullens, Wyoming Co., Enterline and Lainhart (16)	Working miners, random sample, 21 yr and more	44	Not available	More than 80	185	25 (13.5)	10	40	Medium and high rank; low volatility	Pocahontas nos. 3 and 6, Beckley, Sewell
Eastern West Virginia, Richwood, Webster Co., Enterline and Lainhart (16)	Working miners, random sample, 21 yr and more	43	Not available	More than 75	175	11 (6)	2	18	Low and medium rank; medium or high volatility	Sewell, Fire Creek, Pocahontas no. 6
Southern West Virginia, Raleigh Co., Hyatt et al. (17)	Random sample of working miners and ex-miners, 45–55 yr	51.5	52	More than 90	264	121 (46)	19	16	High rank, low volatility	Sewell, Beckley, Fire Creek, Peerless, Pocahontas nos. 3 and 4

a Numbers in parentheses are percentages.

Finally, Hyatt and his colleagues conducted an excellent study in Raleigh County in a random sample of miners aged between 45 and 55 (16). Owing to the criteria for selection, the subjects in this study tended to be somewhat older and to have spent more years underground than those in the other studies. In all these studies again the trend holds true, viz. the higher the rank, the greater the prevalence of radiological abnormalities (Table VII).

Updated Prevalence of Pneumoconiosis in Two States

Late in 1969, the National Coal Study was instituted by the Bureau of Occupational Safety and Health, Public Health Service, to determine prevalence, incidence, and progression of coal workers' pneumoconiosis in the United States. Eventually, some 9,000–10,000 miners in 31 mines in Appalachia, the Midwest, and the Intermountain West will be examined roentgenographically in addition to having been given occupational and medical questionnaires and pulmonary function tests.

Preliminary radiologic data on prevalence of coal workers' pneumoconiosis among bituminous coal miners in five mines in West Virginia and six in Pennsylvania are reported in Table VIII and compared with those from the 1963–1965 prevalence study (6). It is to be noted that different readers have interpreted the roentgenograms and that somewhat different criteria have been utilized for the categorization of pneumoconiosis between the readings in the National Coal Study and the 1963–1965 study. In the National Coal Study, the UICC/Cincinnati Classification of the Pneumoconiosis (8) was used and in the 1963–1965 study, the U. S. Public Health Service modification of the 1958 ILO was utilized (17).

However, by combining those films noted as negative for pneumoconiosis, those suspicious for pneumoconiosis (Category Z), and those with minimal evidence of dust retention (Category 1), the prevalence in 1969–1970 appears to be very similar to that in 1963–1965 in these two states.

Notwithstanding the 5-year interval, there appear to be very similar numbers of men with the various levels (Categories 2 and 3) of simple pneumoconiosis and with complicated Categories A, B, or C pneumoconiosis.

Prevalence of Respiratory Symptoms in Appalachian Miners

So far we have limited ourselves to those conditions which have a direct relationship to the inhalation of coal dust, viz. the various types of CWP. Although CWP can produce both respiratory symptoms and

TABLE VIII

PNEUMOCONIOSIS IN BITUMINOUS-COAL MINERS IN TWO STUDIES IN PENNSYLVANIA AND WEST VIRGINIA

				Percent with Pneumoconiosis[a]				
Study	No. examined	No. pneum. (%)	Suspected pneum. (%)	Simple Cat. 1 (%)	0, Z, and 1 (%)	Simple Cat. 2 (%)	Simple Cat. 3 (%)	Complicated Cat. A, B, & C (%)
National coal study 1969–1970	2709	55.8	—	34.9	90.7	6.8	0.6	1.9
Prevalence 1963–1965 (6)	1702	84.3	5.5	1.7	91.6	5.2	0.4	2.8

[a] Different radiological classifications were used in the two studies (UICC for the 1969–1970 study and ILO for the 1963–1965 study). Hence, comparisons cannot be made for category 0, Z, and 1. In the case of category 2, 3, and complicated pneumoconiosis, it probably is justifiable to compare the percentages although the panel of readers has changed.

respiratory impairment, it is not alone in this. Indeed, since the lungs are capable of responding to insults in a strictly limited manner, it is this self-evident fact that explains why the cornucopia of other respiratory disease cannot be differentiated from CWP on the basis of symptoms and signs alone. The cardinal symptoms of most respiratory diseases are shortness of breath, cough, and sputum; thus, when a cigarette smoking miner presents with these symptoms and an abnormal radiograph compatible with CWP, the physician is seldom able to give a clear-cut answer as to which disease process is responsible for the man's symptoms. Yet since respiratory symptoms occur more frequently in the coal mining population, some effort must be made to separate those symptoms that are a consequence of naturally occurring diseases, e.g., chronic bronchitis, from those symptoms that have an occupational origin. Some consideration must now be given to the occurrence of the respiratory symptoms in the subjects who were included in the Public Health Service study. The prevalence of symptoms was determined by means of a questionnaire, a copy of which is to be found in the appendix of Lainhart's monograph (6).

Cough. Persistent cough in the absence of localized destructive disease of the lungs is the *sine qua non* of chronic bronchitis, and the latter has been shown to be an important disorder among coal mining populations. Although this definition sounds somewhat nonspecific, there are pathological changes found in the condition which make it possible for the severity and extent of chronic bronchitis to be assessed at post mortem or in resected specimens. Clinically, chronic bronchitis may be defined as cough and sputum for at least 3 months in the year for a period of at least 3 years. In Appalachia almost 10% of the working miners and about 24% of the nonworking miners confessed to a persistent productive cough (Table IX) (6).

TABLE IX
HISTORY OF COUGH IN MINERS IN APPALACHIA (6)

Degree of cough	Working miners		Nonworking miners	
	Number	Percent	Number	Percent
No cough or sputum	1810	71.3	561	47.8
Less than persistent productive cough	495	19.5	333	28.4
Persistent productive cough	233	9.2	280	23.8
	2538	100.0	1174	100.0
Unknown cough history	11	—	17	—

TABLE X
HISTORY OF DYSPNEA IN MINERS IN APPALACHIA (6)

	Working miners		Nonworking miners	
Degree of dyspnea	Number	Percent	Number	Percent
None	1209	47.6	174	15.4
Slight	1001	39.4	336	29.7
Moderate	239	9.4	208	18.4
Marked	62	2.5	138	12.2
Severe	28	1.1	275	24.3
	2539	100.0	1,131	100.0
Disabled or unknown dyspnea history	10	—	6[a]	—
	2549	—	1,191	—

[a] Of nonworking miners, 44 were disabled due to noncardiopulmonary causes.

Dyspnea. Shortness of breath, like pain, is a subjective sensation and is therefore difficult to measure. Despite this, it is a most useful indicator of pulmonary insufficiency, and there is a fairly good relationship between the severity of this symptom and the ability to work. In the Public Health Service study, five levels of dyspnea were recognized (Table X) (6). Thus "no" or "slight" dyspnea indicated either no or minimal distress when hurrying on level ground or up a slight hill; "moderate" dyspnea indicated shortness of breath sufficient to cause distress when walking on the level with another person of comparable age who was not distressed, while "marked" and "severe" dyspnea were present when the miner had to stop for breath during the performance of his routine functions, e.g., dressing. Almost 50% of working miners complained of some degree of dyspnea; however, in only 12–13% was it classified as moderate, marked, or severe. There was a relationship between dyspnea, age, and years underground; however, dyspnea seems to be related more to age than to years underground (Table XI and Fig. 6) (6).

Relationship of Respiratory Symptoms to Radiologic Category in Appalachian Miners

The relationship of cough and shortness of breath to radiologic category in the miners who participated in the U. S. Public Health Service study (6) is as follows:

Productive Cough. Persistent cough with phlegm production is associated with those films consistent with pneumoconiosis (Table XII and Fig. 7). Of those working miners with no radiologic evidence of pneu-

TABLE XI

HISTORY OF DYSPNEA BY AGE OF WORKING AND NONWORKING MINERS IN APPALACHIA (6)

Years under-ground	Degree of dyspnea	Less than 35		35–44		45–54		55–64		65 or more		Total	
		Working	Non-working	Working	Non-working	Working	Non-working	Working	Non-working	Working	Non-working	Working	Non-working
0–9	None or slight	190	2	155	15	107	7	48	40	—	—	500	64
	Moderate	7	—	2	3	11	3	8	10	1	—	29	16
	Marked and severe	2 (1.0)[a]	(*)[b]	1 (0.6)	1 (5.3)	1 (1.0)	2 (16.7)	4 (6.7)	21 (29.6)	(*)	(*)	9	26
		199	2	158	19	119	12	60	71	2	2	538	106
10–19	None or slight	103	1	326	26	112	14	10	14	1	2	552	57
	Moderate	2	—	21	9	11	6	3	6	—	—	37	21
	Marked and severe	2 (1.9)	(*)	6 (1.7)	5 (12.5)	3 (2.4)	11 (35.5)	1 (7.1)	17 (45.9)	(*)	(*)	12	33
		107	1	353	40	126	31	14	37	1	2	601	111
20–29	None or slight	1	—	196	4	374	27	60	56	1	5	630	92
	Moderate	—	—	29	2	40	17	10	27	—	—	79	46
	Marked and severe	(*)	—	11 (4.7)	4 (40.0)	13 (3.0)	37 (43.7)	4 (5.4)	57 (40.7)	(*)	*4	28	102
		1	1	236	10	427	81	74	140	1	9	737	240
30–39	None or slight	1		1		253	17	167	161		6	421	184
	Moderate	1		1		32	7	32	68		3	65	78
	Marked and severe	(*)		(*)		15 (5.0)	29 (54.7)	15 (7.0)	151 (39.7)		3 (25.0)	30	183
		2		2		300	53	214	380		12	516	445
40 or more	None or slight					—	1	100	106	3	6	103	113
	Moderate					2	—	27	44	—	3	29	47
	Marked and severe					(*)	(*)	12 (8.6)	68 (31.2)	(*)	1 (10.0)	12	69
						2	1	139	218	3	10	144	229
Unknown history of occupation or dyspnea or disabled												13	60[c]

[a] Numbers in parentheses are percentages.
[b] Asterisk indicates less than 10 persons in grouping.
[c] Of nonworking miners, 44 disabled due to noncardiopulmonary causes.

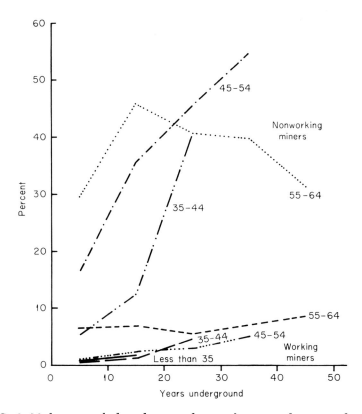

FIG. 6. Moderate, marked, and severe dyspnea by age and years underground among working and nonworking miners.

moconiosis, 8.9% reported persistent productive cough, whereas 13.4% of those with simple pneumoconiotic shadows and 11.9% with complicated pneumoconiosis reported similar symptoms. This association, however, is probably fortuitous and is more likely to be related to the fact that miners with X-ray evidence of the disease are in general older than those with clear films. In this context, the prevalence of chronic bronchitis also increases with advancing age. In general, nonworking miners reported more persistent productive cough, but only those with complicated pneumoconiosis had an increased prevalence of such cough.

Dyspnea. Dyspnea was reported more often in working miners with radiologic evidence of pneumoconiosis than in those classified negative for this condition (Table XIII and Fig. 8). Again this is more likely to be a consequence of the fact that pneumoconiotic miners are, for the most

TABLE XII

History of Cough Related to Roentgenographic Findings of Pneumoconiosis in Miners in Appalachia (6)

	Degree of pneumoconiosis							
	None		Suspect		Simple		Complicated	
Degree of cough	Number	Percent	Number	Percent	Number	Percent	Number	Percent
Working miners:								
No cough or sputum	1530	71.6	98	72.6	113	66.1	53	69.7
Less than persistent productive cough	416	19.5	26	19.3	35	20.5	14	18.4
Persistent productive cough	190	8.9	11	8.1	23	13.4	9	11.9
	2136	100.0	135	100.0	171	100.0	76	100.0
Unknown history or no roentgenogram	31							
Nonworking miners:								
No cough or sputum	428	49.2	37	46.8	49	46.2	41	38.7
Less than persistent productive cough	242	27.8	24	30.4	33	31.1	32	30.2
Persistent productive cough	200	23.0	18	22.8	24	22.7	33	31.1
	870	100.0	79	100.0	106	100.0	106	100.0
Unknown history or no roentgenogram	30							

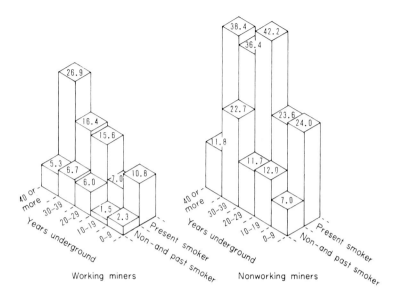

FIG. 7. Persistent productive cough by years underground and cigarette smoking habits among working and nonworking miners.

part, older than their counterparts with clear films. About 3.3% of the working miners whose roentgenograms showed no signs of pneumoconiosis reported marked or severe shortness of breath, whereas 7.0% of those with simple and 5.3% with complicated pneumoconiosis reported this condition. Among the nonworking miners, those men with compli-

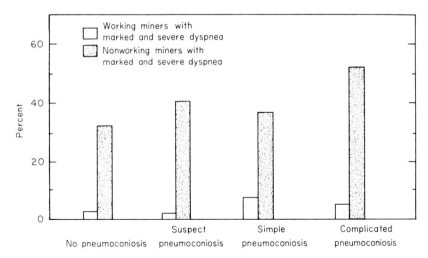

FIG. 8. Dyspnea by degree of pneumoconiosis among working and nonworking miners.

W. S. Lainhart and W. K. C. Morgan

TABLE XIII

HISTORY OF DYSPNEA RELATED TO ROENTGENOGRAPHIC FINDINGS OF PNEUMOCONIOSIS IN MINERS IN APPALACHIA (6)

	Degree of pneumoconiosis							
	None		Suspect		Simple		Complicated	
Degree of dyspnea	Number	Percent	Number	Percent	Number	Percent	Number	Percent
Working miners:								
None or slight	1893	88.6	113	83.7	132	76.7	55	72.3
Moderate	173	8.1	19	14.1	28	16.3	17	22.4
Marked and severe	70	3.3	3	2.2	12	7.0	4	5.3
	2136	100.0	135	100.0	172	100.0	76	100.0
Unknown history or no roentgenogram	30							
Nonworking miners:								
None or slight	401	47.9	33	42.3	46	44.7	24	23.3
Moderate	149	17.8	13	16.7	19	18.4	25	24.3
Marked and severe	287	34.3	32	41.0	38	36.9	54	52.4
	837	100.0	78	100.0	103	100.0	103	100.0
Unknown history or no roentgenogram	70[a]							

[a] Of nonworking miners, 44 disabled due to noncardiopulmonary causes.

cated pneumoconiosis reported a higher incidence of dyspnea (52.4%) than did those whose roentgenograms showed no evidence at all (34.3%).

Appalachian Community Studies

For a variety of reasons it was thought desirable to include a comparable nonmining population in the prevalence study conducted by the U. S. Public Health Service. This allowed a comparison to be made of the respiratory symptoms and respiratory impairment found in a mining and a similar nonmining population. The need for such studies arises from the fact that, as mentioned previously, most respiratory symptoms are nonspecific. Shortness of breath, cough, and sputum may have their origin in a variety of conditions, viz. bronchitis, tuberculosis, and fungous infections. The prevalence of these symptoms is influenced by general factors such as air pollution, cigarette smoking, and individual susceptibility. Thus, the exact role that coal dust plays in producing cough, sputum, and shortness of breath is difficult to determine because of their multifactorial origin. Moreover, with the exception of CWP, American coal miners show little in the way of an excess of deaths from respiratory disease (18). By way of contrast, British coal miners have an excess morbidity and mortality from chronic bronchitis and emphysema. Nonetheless, several studies in both Britain and the United States have shown that coal miners have a lower ventilatory capacity than do men who have never been coal miners. In contrast, a few studies have failed to bear out this impression (19). To lessen the effects of differing environments, the U. S. Public Health Service sought two communities in which the potential male employees had a more or less random choice of entering either coal mining or another, nondusty occupation. The ideal community would be one in which the earnings of those in the nondusty occupation were roughly the same as those of the coal miners, so that socioeconomic and educational factors such as the availability and utilization of medical care would be roughly comparable. Needless to say, this sort of situation is very infrequent. Additional characteristics sought were that (1) the industries should be stable and fairly long established so that a major portion of the labor force had been employed in the industry for several years, (2) both types of worker should be living in the same section or area of the town so that there were common social and other activities, and (3) the communities should be political entities so that demographic data would be available. Under these circumstances, it was felt that most environmental influences would be the same for both occupations and if the two groups were found to differ, it would be reasonable to assume that the occupational environment was responsible.

The two communities selected were Richwood and Mullens (15). The former is a community of about 5000 and is situated in east central West Virginia. Its two main occupations are coal mining and lumbering. Mullens is situated in the southern part of West Virginia, and its economy depends mainly on coal mining and on the railroad. Extensive marshalling yards are present in the town. As already indicated earlier in the chapter, there was the additional difference that the coal mined in Mullens is of higher rank than that mined in Richwood. Incomes tended to be higher in Mullens than in Richwood. There were relatively more elderly persons in Richwood, and the educational level attained was somewhat less. Cigarette smoking did not differ in the two communities. Residents of Mullens had more respiratory symptoms, in particular dyspnea, than did those from Richwood. In both areas more than 50% of the working male population had spent time in the coal mines. The educational level of the coal miners was lower than that of nonminers in Mullens, but not in Richwood.

The percentage of participation in both communities was excellent. The subjects in the study had the aforementioned questionnaire (6) administered to them, a standard chest film was taken, and the forced vital capacity was measured. To confirm that any observed differences between coal miners and other manual workers were the consequence of occupational exposure, it was decided to examine the wives of both occupational groups. If the nonoccupational environment was to differ for the two occupations, it would be exected that the wives of the two groups would also differ since they would be exposed to the same nonoccupational influences along with their husbands. On the other hand if the occupational environment accounted for any difference found, then the wives of the two groups would be expected to resemble each other.

Results of the Mullens Examinations

Seven hundred and five subjects between the age of 21 and 64 were examined. This represents somewhat over 85% of the total of 825 who were asked to participate. Table XIV shows the relevant data. Percentages related to respiratory symptoms, and previous histories of pneumonia and pleurisy, are adjusted to the age and educational-level distribution of miners. Percentages for respiratory symptoms of wives of miners had been adjusted by the direct method to the age and cigarette distribution of the wives of nonminers. The mean height of miners was almost an inch less than that of nonminers. It is evident from the table that in all subjects there was a clearcut relationship between cigarette smoking and respiratory symptoms.

The miners on the whole reported more cough and sputum than did the nonminers. Somewhat surprisingly this effect seemed to be carried over into the wives of the coal miners, and miners' wives admitted sputum production more frequently than the wives of the railroad workers. The same trend was apparent in regard to dyspnea.

Radiological evidence of pneumoconiosis was almost entirely confined to coal miners. Since the radiologists reporting the films were not aware of the man's occupation, any form of bias related to a knowledge of the man's job can be excluded from the results.

When the results of spirometric measurements are compared for each group, it is apparent that miners have a lower ventilatory capacity than do the nonminers. On the other hand, and somewhat surprisingly in view of the increased prevalence of respiratory symptoms, miners' wives did not show a reduction in the FEV_1/FVC % or other tests of ventilatory capacity when compared to the wives of railroad workers.

RESULTS OF THE RICHWOOD EXAMINATIONS

Of 803 persons invited to participate, 609 (74.7%) did so. This is a slightly less satisfactory response than in Mullens.

The mean age of the miners examined was slightly lower than for the nonminers. The miners tended to be lighter, shorter, and to have more cough and sputum. They were reported more wheezy. Dyspnea was reported more often in the miners and their wives than in the nonminers and their wives.

As in Mullens, there was a definite relationship between the radiologic findings and occupation. In contrast to Mullens, the ventilatory capacity of the Richwood miners did not differ from that of the nonmining group.

DISCUSSION OF COMMUNITY STUDIES

The finding in Mullens that not only miners, but also their wives, had more respiratory symptoms than the comparable control groups was not unexpected in view of the British studies (19, 20). These findings have been used as an argument against the hypothesis that coal dust produces a form of industrial bronchitis (4). Nonetheless, this conclusion has been disputed since although respiratory symptoms occur more commonly in miners' wives than in nonminers' wives, the concomitant and associated reduction in ventilatory capacity that is found in the miners is not present in their spouses.

On the other hand, an explanation for these findings may be present in the nonoccupational environment. The excess respiratory symptoms found in the miners' wives may be influenced by their educational attain-

TABLE XIV
Selected Results of Medical Examinations from Appalachia Study

Medical examination item	Mullens, men Miners	Mullens, men Nonminers	Richwood, men Miners	Richwood, men Nonminers	Mullens, wives Miners	Mullens, wives Nonminers	Richwood, wives Miners	Richwood, wives Nonminers
Invited for examination	225	224	225	224	191	185	196	158
Actually examined	185	194	175	153	163	163	156	116
Percentage examined	82.2	86.8	77.8	68.0	85.3	88.1	79.6	73.4
Mean age, years	43.9	43.8	42.8	43.8	40.3	41.0	39.0	42.0
Mean height, inches	68.3	69.1	69.1	69.4	63.3	63.5	64.5	64.3
Mean weight, pounds	166.4	178.1	164.8	166.5	141.5	142.8	151.0	142.3
Cigarette smoking, pack year	23.8	25.0	22.4	27.8	9.7	6.1	8.5	9.1
Cough and phlegm:								
Any cough	49 (26.5)[a]	31 (17.4)	30 (18.7)	31 (20.2)	21 (10.0)	16 (10.0)	17 (10.8)	9 (7.7)
>3 mo, >3 yr[b]	26 (14.0)	14 (8.9)	23 (14.1)	20 (13.0)	13 (6.4)	7 (4.2)	9 (5.7)	7 (6.0)
Any phlegm production	47 (25.4)	37 (21.1)	18 (11.1)	20 (13.0)	23 (11.7)	11 (7.0)	11 (7.0)	5 (4.3)
>3 mo, >3 yr	28 (15.1)	26 (14.7)	14 (8.9)	14 (9.1)	11 (5.3)	2	5 (3.2)	4
Wheezing:								
Any wheezing	103 (55.7)	89 (49.8)	91 (52.5)	67 (43.7)	56 (34.0)	44 (27.0)	47 (30.1)	37 (31.8)
With colds only	61 (33.0)	57 (32.6)	50 (28.2)	38 (24.8)	27 (17.2)	30 (18.4)	31 (19.8)	25 (21.5)
Other times too	42 (22.7)	32 (17.2)	41 (24.5)	29 (18.9)	29 (16.7)	14 (8.6)	16 (10.3)	12 (10.3)
Dyspnea:								
Disabled, not cardiopulmonary	10	4	1	1	2	2	1	0
Not disabled	174	189	155	152	160	157	155	116
Grade 3 (moderate) or worse	42 (24.1)	27 (14.5)	23 (14.8)	13 (8.5)	37 (22.0)	20 (12.7)	25 (16.1)	13 (11.2)
Grade 5 (severe)	8 (5.0)	7 (4.6)	7 (4.6)	7 (4.6)	13 (7.4)	4	6 (3.9)	2

History of pneumonia:								
Any history	70 (38.0)	49 (26.8)	68 (38.8)	48 (31.4)	53 (32.5)	35 (21.4)	54 (34.6)	28 (24.1)
Before age 18 only	28 (15.0)	19 (9.9)	18 (10.9)	21 (13.7)	22 (13.5)	18 (11.0)	17 (10.9)	12 (10.3)
18 or later	42 (23.0)	30 (18.3)	50 (28.6)	27 (17.6)	31 (19.0)	17 (10.4)	27 (23.7)	16 (13.8)
Single episode	33 (18.0)	25 (14.4)	33 (18.8)	23 (15.0)	24 (15.0)	17 (10.4)	28 (17.9)	14 (12.1)
Multiple episodes	9 (5.0)	16 (7.8)	17 (9.7)	4	7 (4.3)	0	9 (5.8)	2
History of pleurisy:								
Any history	36 (19.4)	21 (9.7)	23 (13.1)	8 (5.2)	25 (15.3)	27 (16.5)	13 (8.3)	16 (13.8)
Before age 18	4	2	2	0	6 (4.0)	2	2	6 (5.2)
18 or later	32 (17.2)	19 (8.7)	21 (12.0)	8 (5.2)	19 (12.0)	25 (15.3)	11 (7.1)	10 (8.6)
Single episode	22 (12.0)	14 (7.0)	17 (9.7)	7 (4.6)	16 (10.0)	19 (12.0)	8 (5.1)	9 (7.8)
Multiple episodes	10 (5.4)	5	4	1	3	6 (4.0)	3	1
Roentgenographic findings:								
Definite pneumoconiosis	25 (13.5)	2	11 (6.3)	1	0	2	0	0
Suspect pneumoconiosis	10 (5.4)	2	6 (3.4)	2	0	2	1	0
Simple pneumoconiosis	15 (8.1)	2	9 (5.1)	1	0	2	0	0
Complicated pneumoconiosis	10 (5.4)	0	2	0	0	0	0	0
Forced expiratory volumes:								
FEV_1 (liters/second)	2.98	3.18	3.29	3.28	2.32	2.33	2.52	2.46
Total FEV (liters/second)	4.08	4.15	4.32	4.29	2.94	2.93	3.09	3.05
FEV_1/FEV (percent)	72.6	76.3	75.9	76.4	78.6	78.7	81.3	80.8

[a] Number in parentheses is percentage of the total number of examinees from whom information was available. Percentages for respiratory symptoms among male nonminers and wives of coal miners have been adjusted. Percentages were not calculated for less than five cases.

[b] Present most days for more than 3 months a year and for more than 3 years.

ment since there is some evidence to suggest that the lower the educational level of a person, the more likely he or she is to complain of symptoms. Moreover, there is a natural reluctance on the part of the better educated person to admit to cough and sputum. Alternatively the miners' wives may undergo a form of psychological contamination from hearing and seeing their husbands constantly coughing and spitting. A third possibility lies in the fact that miners' bronchitis may have an infectious origin which is transmitted to their wives.

The causes for disparate findings in the miners in Mullens as compared to Richwood remains a mystery. There is little reason to believe that selection can account for the differences. Although the work histories taken in Richwood were shorter, this in itself was not of sufficient magnitude to explain the difference in ventilatory capacity. The other possible explanations may be related to differences in air pollution and in the coal mined in the two communities. In this connection, Mullens is more polluted and has coal fields of a higher rank. Further work on these problems is necessary.

REFERENCES

1. Carpenter, R. B., et al. (1956). Brit. J. Ind. Med. 13, 166.
2. Higgins, I. T. T., et al. (1956). Brit. Med. J. 2, 904.
3. Enterline, P. (1967). Arch. Environ. Health 14, 189.
4. Medical Research Council (1966). Brit. Med. J. 1, 101.
5. Lainhart, W. S. (1969). J. Occup. Med. 11, 399.
6. Lainhart, W. S., et al. (1969). Pub. Health Ser. Publ. 2000.
7. Pendergrass, E. P., et al. (1965). Arch. Environ. Health 10, 776.
8. Hart, P. D. A., and Aslett, E. A. (1942). Med. Res. Counc. Gt. Brit. Spec. Rep. Ser. 243.
9. Morgan, W. K. C. (1968). Amer. Rev. Resp. Dis. 98, 306.
10. American Society for Testing and Materials, Philadelphia, Pa. (1967). "Standard Specifications for Classification of Coal by Rank." Standard Doc. 388-66, Pt. 19.
11. McBride, W. W., Pendergrass, E. P., and Lieben, J. J. (1966). J. Occup. Med. 8, 365.
12. Lieben, J., Pendergrass, E. P., and McBride, W. W. (1961). J. Occup. Med. 3, 493.
13. McBride, W. W., Pendergrass, E. P., and Lieben, J. J. (1963). J. Occup. Med. 5, 376.
14. Higgins, I. T. T., et al. (1968). Brit. J. Ind. Med. 25, 165.
15. Enterline, P. E., and Lainhart, W. S. (1967). Amer. J. Pub. Health 57, 484.
16. Hyatt, R. E., Kistin, A. D., and Mahan, T. K. (1964). Amer. Rev. Resp. Dis. 89, 387.
17. UICC Committee, Cincinnati, Ohio (1970). Chest 58, 57.
18. Enterline, P. E. (1964). Amer. J. Pub. Health 54, 758.
19. Higgins, I. T. T., et al. (1959). Brit. J. Ind. Med. 16, 255.
20. Higgins, I. T. T., and Cochrane, A. L. (1961). Brit. J. Ind. Med. 18, 93.

4

Symptomatology

Murray B. Hunter

When coal miners become aware that they may have a chronic disease of the lung, their symptoms, save one, are indistinguishable from those of chronic pulmonary disease seen in the general nonmining population. The one specific symptom that identifies the coal miner is melanoptysis, the production of black or coal-flecked sputum. Melanoptysis, however, does not necessarily denote radiographic pneumoconiosis inasmuch as it is common to miners who inhale coal dust in quantity and who cough. Melanoptysis is not related to X-ray category and is seen equally in men with and without dust opacification on the X ray. Perhaps the only symptom that is truly unique to coal miners ill from pneumoconiosis and that is reproducible in no other disease state is the production of liquid inky sputum seen in complicated pneumoconiosis when the fibrotic areas undergo avascular necrosis and their centers cavitate.

Other symptoms of which significant numbers of coal miners complain are dyspnea, cough, usually with sputum production, wheezing, frequent chest illnesses necessitating loss of time from work or a period of bed rest, and chest pains, not attributable to coronary artery disease. Miners and exminers with the above noted symptoms, either alone or in combination, often indicate that their symptomatology is aggravated in inclement weather, worse in the winter, and if wheezing is present it is maximal in the early morning hours of 4 to 6 a.m. The entire constellation of dyspnea, productive cough, episodic wheezing, frequent chest illness, and aggravation by inclement weather has been termed the "respiratory symptom complex" (1). Some symptomatic miners have the full syndrome, but others experience only one or two of the above symptom categories. The most frequent single symptom of which miners complain is dyspnea; this is often seen independently of other components of the full complex. In any event, it is natural for the symptomatic miner to assume that his difficulties are caused by his occupation. As a general rule, however, that assumption is shared by his physician and by the separate state and federal compensation agencies only when the X ray demonstrates dust opacification. The lack of concurrence between what the symptomatic miner assumes about the cause and effect relationship of occupation to symptoms and what the medical and legal professions assume in this regard is responsible for much of the tension that exists in the coal fields today.

A multiplicity of studies has been undertaken, first in Britain and more recently in the United States, that are designed to test the relationships between symptomatology and duration of exposure to dust, age, X-ray category of pneumoconiosis, tobacco smoking, ventilatory function, oxygen transport (in a few studies), and socioenvironmental factors. The epidemiologic studies thus far undertaken have attempted to answer some or all of the following questions:

1. What is the relationship between the number and duration of symptoms reported in coal miners to objective tests of pulmonary function?

2. Do miners and exminers have more symptoms of chronic respiratory tract disease and impaired lung function than men of similar age who have never worked in the mines but who lived in the same area?

3. Do miners and exminers with radiographic pneumoconiosis have more symptoms of chronic respiratory disease and impaired lung function than miners and exminers without radiographic pneumoconiosis? If so, how much more?

4. What is the effect of other known pulmonary irritants, such as cigarette smoke, on symptoms and impairment in coal miners?

The evidence obtained from these separate surveys is uniform with respect to some relationships and contradictory in others. The relationship on which there seems to be the greatest concordance is that between symptoms and ventilatory function. With increase in the duration and number of symptoms, ventilatory function tends to decline proportionately, a finding that belies the assertion of some (2, 3) that there is a very large input of respiratory neurosis into the totality of symptomatology in working and retired coal miners. On the contrary, the relationship between symptoms and radiographic pneumoconiosis is a complex one in which there is a great deal of observer variation. Answers to the above questions cannot be assayed without reference to both epidemiologic and clinical data specific for each symptom as well as for the full respiratory symptom complex.

Dyspnea

At the moment in time when miners become patients on a regular basis and seek treatment, advice or advocacy from a physician, their principal complaint is effort dyspnea and their description of their level of dyspnea is equivalent to grade 2 or 3 dyspnea of Fletcher (4). Most systematic surveys of respiratory symptoms in coal miners indicate that miners who develop symptoms begin to complain of effort dyspnea, typically at ages 50–55, after 25–30 years of underground mining. Grading of dyspnea is essential to precision in symptom analysis as a guide to assessment of progression of disease and as a means of standardizing symptom statements to facilitate comparison between studies of different groups of miners. Fletcher's original questionnaire (4) identified five grades of dyspnea as follows:

Breathlessness (average in last winter)
Grade 1. Are you ever troubled by breathlessness except on strenuous exertion?
Grade 2. (If yes.) Are you short of breath when hurrying on the level or walking up a slight hill?
Grade 3. (If yes.) Do you have to walk slower than most people on the level? Do you have to stop after a mile or so (or after ¼ hour) on the level at your own pace?
Grade 4. (If yes to either.) Do you have to stop for breath after walking about 100 yd (or after a few minutes) on the level?
Grade 5. (If yes.) Are you too breathless to leave the house, or are you breathless after undressing?

The Fletcher questions were modified slightly in the Raleigh County, W. Va., study of respiratory symptomatology in coal miners (5), modifications that were also employed in the U. S. Public Health Service study of pneumoconiosis (6). The modification is as follows:

If the subject answers "No" to all of the following questions, the classification is grade 1. The other grades depend on the last of the questions to which the answer is "Yes."
Grade 2. Do you ever get short of breath hurrying on the level or walking up a slight hill?

Grade 3. Do you get short of breath walking with people your own age on a level or do you walk slower than they do?

Grade 4. Do you have to stop because of shortness of breath while walking at your own speed on the level?

Grade 5. Are you breathless on washing or after dressing?

In most studies where the term breathlessness is used alone, without specific reference to grading, perusal of the text indicates that most authors begin to use the term breathlessness or dyspnea as a symptomatic statement equivalent to grade 3.

It has been shown that assessment of symptomatology carried out in this fashion carries with it a high degree of reliability on repeat questioning by the same observer and a minimum of skew when the same questions are put by different observers (7, 8).

Many miners live in hilly communities and they may first become aware of dyspnea when going to and from the road or mailbox rather than on the job. Most miners with grade-3 dyspnea complain of generalized lassitude as well as of a curious complaint of leg pain or cramping in the thigh or calf musculature, not accountable for on the basis of impairment of the peripheral circulation. Orthopnea is not an accompaniment of the dyspnea seen in coal miners unless there is coexistent congestive failure. Those patients with early morning bronchospasm report that they often experience wheezing or chest tightness while sitting up or getting out of bed. Dyspnea tends to be slowly progressive after its appearance although a few miners report improvement upon removal from dust. This is not accompanied by evidence of better lung function and probably reflects a lower breathing requirement for ordinary day-to-day activities after retirement.

In clinical practice, few miners are seen with grade-5 dyspnea. Those who are living at this level either have severe emphysema, with or without dust opacification on the X ray or large areas of massive fibrosis on the film. In the Raleigh County, W. Va., study (5), those miners graded as experiencing dyspnea while washing or dressing had a ratio of residual volume to lung capacity (RV/TLC) of 47%, whereas miners at all other grades of dyspnea had near normal RV/TLC of 35–39%. This observation tends to support the view of Motley (9) that over the whole range of pneumoconiosis, the best index of disability is the expression of residual volume as a percentage of total lung capacity, the inference being that dyspnea in pneumoconiosis is caused by emphysema. Gilson and Hugh-Jones (10), expressing the view that both tests are highly predictive, believe that the maximum breathing capacity best correlates with dyspnea in coal miners.

While breathlessness is commonly seen in coal miners as a single symptom, cyanosis is rare unless there are multiple symptoms, particularly wheezing or chest tightness and productive cough. It is virtually impossible to divide symptomatic coal miners with or without dust opacification on the X ray into "pink puffers" (anatomic emphysema, underweight, small hearts, scant sputum, large lungs, no history of heart failure, and near normal blood gases) and "blue bloaters" (arterial desaturation, elevated hematocrit, hypercapnea, larger volumes of sputum, little anatomical emphysema, under ventilation, and heavier body weights). When either type is seen in near pure form and with manifest high-grade impairment, one is not impressed with a particular relationship to dust concentration on the film.

Not infrequently in clinical practice, miners are encountered who complain bitterly of dyspnea of effort but whose ventilatory function tests are normal. These individuals may become the objects of personality inventory, but it has been suggested by Rasmussen (11) in a study of non-smoking coal miners that dyspnea in the presence of normal ventilation is related to impairment in oxygen transfer. His views deserve to be quoted in some detail for they represent perhaps the most extreme estimate of the deleterious effects of coal mining upon health.

"Impairment in oxygen transfer is almost always encountered among our symptomatic miners. This finding is more frequent than ventilatory insufficiency among those miners complaining of significant effort dyspnea. There is, however, a rather poor correlation between the severity of symptoms and the magnitude of the gas transfer insufficiency. In some miners who admit to no significant effort dyspnea and who also exhibit no intolerance to moderate to heavy exercise, mild impairment of oxygen transfer has been noted. These subjects exhibit increased $(A-a)O_2$ gradients, slight hypoxia, reduced fractional carbon monoxide uptake, and often slightly subnormal steady state diffusing capacities. In a very small number of miners studied serially at two to three and one-half year intervals, oxygen transfer impairment has appeared, even though the subjects deny definite symptoms and exercise tolerance remains normal. We believe that oxygen transfer impairment may be one preclinical physiologic abnormality, in some coal miners."

Most respiratory physiologists who have studied gas transfer in coal miners do not share this impression, and the generally accepted viewpoint has been that deficits in gas transfer are largely limited to complicated pneumoconiosis (10). Recently, Lyons and co-workers were able to demonstrate reduced diffusing capacity in subjects with the pinhead but not the nodular type of simple pneumoconiosis (12).

A second explanation for the coexistence of dyspnea and normal ventilatory function is the observation (12a) that tests of ventilatory function employed in most laboratories do not measure resistance in peripheral or small airways, sites which on the basis of pathologic findings in coal miners' lungs seem likely to be sites of predilection for difficulties of function.

Dyspnea and the X Ray

Radiographic pneumoconiosis at all levels of severity is compatible with absence of symptoms. Fletcher (13) described a local sprint champion whose X ray showed progressive massive fibrosis. Martin (14), in a pioneer study of coalworkers' pneumoconiosis in West Virginia, concluded that "the chest X-ray is virtually worthless as a means of estimating disability." It is not suggested that most men with progressive massive fibrosis (PMF) are free of dyspnea. Dyspnea in PMF appears to be a function of the area of involvement on the P-A X ray of the chest and is manifest usually only after the total area of involvement is in excess of 20 cm^2 (15, 15a). With simple pneumoconiosis there is even less relationship of the X ray to dyspnea from the data secured in most studies, although a few report increase in dyspnea with an increasing degree of simple pneumoconiosis (16, 17). A consensus view would appear to be that there is little correlation until category-3 simple pneumoconiosis is reached, by which time most studies report increases in dyspnea and in the ventilatory function tests which correlate with dyspnea (FEV$_1$ and/or MBC).

Some idea of the conceptual difficulties which are created by these complex relationships may be obtained when the actual percentages and numbers of individuals with symptoms and with positive X rays are considered. Pneumoconiosis prevalence shows wide variation between different studies with a low of 11% cited by Higgins (18) for Marion County, W. Va., 23–57% in three United Kingdom communities (1, 6, 17, 19, 20), and 46% for miners aged 45–55 in southern West Virginia (5). If half of a given cohort of coal miners have a positive X ray and half are symptomatic (approximately the number encountered in many surveys) and the relationship between symptoms and the X ray is totally random, then one miner in four will have symptoms and a positive X ray, one in four will have symptoms and a negative X ray, one in four will have no symptoms and a positive X ray, and the other will have neither symptoms nor a positive X ray. In clinical practice, this hypothetical model comes remarkably close to the empiric observation of many physicians practicing in the field.

There seems to be little question from epidemiologic studies that miners and exminers have more respiratory symptoms than nonmining men of the same age, living in the same communities. The magnitude of this difference is small in some places, but this observation is consistent with the clinical estimates of physicians living in coal mining communities who treat both miners and nonminers.

Cough and Sputum; Bronchitis

Cough is present in 25–45% of working miners with radiographic pneumoconiosis and in approximately 50% of retired miners with radiographic pneumoconiosis (1, 5, 6, 17, 19–21). It was present in 49% of miners without radiographic pneumoconiosis in the Raleigh County, W. Va., study (5). Cough is generally productive of sputum, described as milky, gray, white or clear, and often coal-flecked ("bug dust"). With superimposition of episodic infective bronchitis, sputum becomes yellow, green, or "thick." With each such episode of superimposed infective bronchitis, cough becomes aggravated and sputum production increases. Episodic bronchitis may be associated with fever and increased dyspnea, and sometimes it may be the cause of the onset of acute congestive heart failure, usually biventricular, rather than classically right-sided. Some coal miners report the onset of chronic dyspnea as having followed an acute, apparently infectious chest illness, either a frank pneumonia, or acute bronchitis ("flu").

In some miners cough is so persistent and sputum so copious that the diagnosis of bronchiectasis is entertained, but clubbing is rarely seen in coal miners without obvious cause, and when miners are subjected to bronchoscopy or bronchography, bronchiectasis is exceedingly rare (22).

Hemoptysis is rare as part of coalworkers' pneumoconiosis, and when seen, nonoccupational disease such as carcinoma of the lung, tuberculosis (considered occupational when associated with silicosis), pulmonary embolism, or bronchiectasis must be considered first. Occasionally with severe PMF, blood will be produced along with heavily coal-contaminated sputum.

Asthma as the first symptom preceding cough or dyspnea almost certainly rules out occupationally related disease. "Miner's asthma" is cough, sputum, and dyspnea first and asthma later. When wheezing is the first symptom to be recorded in time, nonoccupational allergy is found. There are no proven allergenic properties in coal dust, and miners do not report a syndrome of Monday morning bronchospasm as has been observed in textile workers.

Miners who do wheeze report their "tightness" in association with intercurrent respiratory infections or in bad weather. Aggravation of chest symptomatology in bad weather has been accepted in the United Kingdom and in the United States as part of the respiratory symptom complex, but the association has never been put to the test of validity and may reflect an intrusion of folk associations into clinical science.

Although there are still differences between the definition of chronic bronchitis preferred in the United Kingdom (23) and in the United States (24), it has become clear that in all societies the presence of a chronic productive cough not explainable by specific infectious or infiltrative disease is the essential clinical criterion of chronic bronchitis. Its pathologic expression is hypertrophy of the mucous glands and goblet cells of the bronchi and bronchioles. It has been more precisely defined clinically as chronic, productive cough on most days (especially in the winter months) for at least two years. In practice the average individual with chronic bronchitis may not regard himself as ill unless and until he has developed, with his bronchitis, chronic airway obstruction and thus associated dyspnea of effort. Fletcher et al. (4) divided bronchitis into two grades: Grade 1 comprises individuals who produce sputum only on rising or only later in the day; grade 2 comprises those who produce sputum both on rising and throughout the day. Higgins et al. (25) has added to the definition (besides persistent sputum and cough) a chest illness causing loss of work or an acute episode lasting three weeks but not necessarily causing loss of work or bed rest. Most studies of bronchitis have confirmed the prevalence of this type of symptomatology to be greater among coal miners than in the control nonmining populations. The magnitude of excess bronchitis for coal miners is variable, as it is with other chest symptomatology, slight in some areas and considerable in others. Magnitudes of prevalence of chronic bronchitis among coal miners vary from 16–43% among working miners (5, 6, 8, 12a, 17, 20, 21, 25, 26). Comparable ranges for nonmining population studies are 5–25%. A curious by-product of bronchitis research has been the finding that in several studies (6, 19, 20) miners' wives had higher bronchitis rates than the wives of nonminers. The point has yet to be explained. It may reveal only proneness on the part of miners' wives to answer the bronchitis questionnaire in an affirmative fashion. This explanation is appealing to those who daily treat miners' wives and do not encounter any unusual frequency of chronic chest disease in them. Other tenable explanations are that bronchitis might be caused in part by community-wide exposure to airborne products of bituminous coal mining or that a bronchitis producing agent (coal dust?) is brought home by the miner on his skin or clothing.

Study of the time sequence of development of symptoms may be of value in understanding the relationship between environment and disease and the effect of the development of one symptom upon another. In contrast to the sequence in the nonmining population where cough generally precedes dyspnea, Gilson and Hugh-Jones (10) reported that in 41 out of 50 miners with radiographic pneumoconiosis breathlessness antedates cough. In clinical experience smoking habits appear to govern the time sequence of symptom production, smokers tending to cough earlier than nonsmokers. In this connection some data from the National Coal Board Field Research (Table I) are of interest (27). About 20,000 miners in all coal-mining regions were given a questionnaire of respiratory symptoms and smoking habits. Each figure indicates the average age at which 20% of the men in each category developed a particular symptom. It would appear that radiographic pneumoconiosis and smoking have a similar and additive effect in inducing the early development of bronchitic symptoms.

In addition to earlier development of symptoms, smoking coal miners report more symptoms than do nonsmoking miners and their function tests tend to be poorer. Earlier surveys indicated an incidence of nonsmoking of 10–15% among coal miners, but this figure is certainly on the rise at present. In general, men with poorer ventilatory function tend to become exsmokers. "Cigarette cough" alone will not provoke nonsmoking in individuals addicted to tobacco, but the development of sputum production, wheezing, and dyspnea tends to provoke men to give up smoking. As a result, in large-scale surveys, exsmokers might be expected to have the poorest function and the most symptoms. This expectation is borne out in some of the studies cited but not in others. Too often it is assumed (21) that coughing, in turn induced in part by smoking, plays a beneficial role in helping to clear the lungs and respiratory passages of excessive secretions and furthers the clearance mechanism for coal dust. Were this so, there would be an inverse correlation between radiographic pneumoconiosis, on the one hand, and smoking and coughing on the other. Such an inverse correlation does not in fact obtain. Patients who persist with severe chronic and persistent coughing with sputum production are the ones whose clinical status deteriorates the most rapidly. When coughing is in part controlled by cessation of smoking and other measures favorable to bronchial hygiene, the clinical status of the patient improves.

Answers to the questions posed above are summarized as follows. In some instances answers are firm and in others tentative.

1. On the relationship of symptoms to function: Symptoms are predictive of function, with the greatest concordance being that between dyspnea and function.

2. Comparison of miners and nonminers: Miners, irrespective of the presence of radiographic pneumoconiosis, have a higher prevalence of all symptoms than comparable nonminers, and they have lower average pulmonary function as well.

TABLE I

Age Estimates for Smoking Status by X-Ray Category, by Symptoms
(20% of Sample with 95% Confidence Limits All Regions)[a]

Category of subject	Symptom					
	Cough	Sputum	Breathlessness	Wheeze	Weather	Chest illness
Smokers						
Cat. 0	45.9 (45.2, 46.5)	47.1 (46.3, 47.9)	50.5 (50.0, 51.0)	43.6 (43.0, 44.2)	44.7 (44.1, 45.3)	48.7 (47.7, 49.7)
Cat. 1+	36.3 (32.5, 39.0)	36.2 (31.2, 39.5)	38.9 (36.7, 40.6)	27.8 (21.5, 32.0)	25.7 (18.9, 30.3)	40.5 (36.4, 43.2)
Nonsmokers						
Cat. 0	67.0 (62.2, 74.0)	77.3[b] (67.8, 94.9)	57.1 (52.2, 59.5)	54.6 (52.5, 57.1)	54.0 (51.9, 56.6)	57.4 (53.9, 62.3)
Cat. 1+	55.3 (51.3, 61.1)	52.0 (47.6, 56.2)	43.9 (39.6, 46.7)	44.2 (37.1, 48.0)	41.8 (34.7, 45.6)	44.8 (33.5, 49.6)
Exsmokers						
Cat. 0	56.5 (53.9, 59.8)	54.3 (51.3, 58.3)	52.2 (50.6, 53.9)	47.1 (45.2, 48.8)	47.9 (46.0, 49.8)	46.0 (43.3, 48.5)
Cat. 1+	44.2 (27.0, 51.3)	40.0	40.5 (31.3, 45.1)	39.7 (28.3, 44.8)	29.2 (26.7, 39.0)	29.7

[a] From J. Rogan (27).
[b] Extrapolated value.

3. Comparison of miners with and without radiographic pneumo-coniosis: Studies, apparently equally well designed, have provided some-what discordant answers to this question. A balanced view, tentatively offered, is that radiographic pneumoconiosis may have a modest aggra-vating effect upon symptoms and function. This effect is at best minimal in categories 1 and 2 simple pneumoconiosis, modest at category 3 and in complicated pneumoconiosis with a small area of involvement, and definitely appreciable only with complicated pneumoconiosis involving large areas of the lungs.

4. Cigarette smoking, symptoms, and impairment: Miners who smoke have more symptoms, especially symptoms of bronchitis, than nonsmok-ing miners. Their symptoms appear at an earlier age and they have poorer function than nonsmoking miners. Smoking, however, does not account for the differences between miners and nonminers (27a). Total lifetime tobacco smoke inhalation does not account for the positive correlation between years worked underground and impairment of pulmonary function (5).

Clinical and epidemiologic studies of the host–dose relationship in underground coal mining are of value only if they help to illuminate the nature of the disease specific to coal miners and to point the way to fur-ther study and action designed to facilitate prevention. Both kinds of data suggest hypotheses about the relationship of occupation to the health of the underground miner, which, while not representing totally inescap-able conclusions, nevertheless provide a framework for further thought and study. It is conceivable and suggested by symptom analysis and by radiographic analysis of large numbers of miners that mining affects the miner in two separate, although possibly parallel, ways. The first effect is responsible for dust opacification on the X ray, and for purposes of clarity, the agent or agents responsible for it may be termed the "X-ray opacification factor." Another effect of underground coal mining upon the worker is the production of respiratory symptoms. The agent or agents responsible for this effect may be termed the "symptom-producing factor." The X-ray opacification factor is certainly coal dust, and its effects are expressed in men who do all varieties of underground work, both at the coal face and in haulage and maintenance operations. The symptom-producing factor in underground coal mining may also be coal dust, or something in coal dust, or it may be something entirely apart from coal dust. A theoretical system, assuming that it is something other than coal dust, is consistent with the existing data on the subject and is consistent with clinical experience as well. After the effects of the X-ray opacifica-tion factor in coal mining are felt for a long enough time and in quantity sufficient to produce a category-3 or greater X ray, the individual who has sustained the accumulation of too much dust is rendered thereby more susceptible to the effects of the symptom-producing factor. In the case of far-advanced progressive massive fibrosis the X-ray opacification factor alone may be responsible for all the observed phenomena. Dust alone, when it reaches a critical mass in the lungs, may be responsible for PMF with all of its attendant manifestations. However, in most symptomatic miners the effects of either the symptom-producing factor, operating alone or in combination with what produces high-grade X-ray change, are responsible for the total clinical picture as seen by the physician. Whatever the symptom-producing factor is, it is located underground, and while its expression may be facilitated by smoking, air pollution, and general socioenvironmental factors, it is basically either part or a by-product of underground mining operations.

REFERENCES

1. Ashford, J. R., Brown, S., Morgan, D. C., and Rae, S. (1968). *Amer. Rev. Resp. Dis.* **97**, 810.
2. Nestmann, R. H. (1956). *W. Va. Med. J.* **52**, 149.
3. Ross, W. D., Miller, L. H., Leet, H. H., and Princi, F. (1954). *J. Amer. Med. Ass.* **156**, 484.
4. Fletcher, C. M., Elmes, P. C., Fairbairn, A. S., and Wood, C. H. (1959). *Brit. Med. J.* **2**, 257.
5. Hyatt, R. E., Kistin, A. D., and Mahan, T. K. (1964). *Amer. Rev. Resp. Dis.* **89**, 387.
6. Lainhart, W. S., Doyle, H. N., Enterline, P. E., Henschel, A., and Kendrick, M. A. "Pneumoconiosis in Appalachian Bituminous Coal Miners." U. S. Department of Health, Education, and Welfare, Public Health Service.
7. Cochrane, A. L., Chapman, P. J., and Oldham, P. D. (1951). *Lancet* **1**, 1007.
8. Fairbairn, A. S., Wood, C. H., and Fletcher, C. M. (1959). *Brit. J. Prev. Soc. Med.* **13**, 175.
9. Motley, H. L., and Lang, L. P. (1948). *Amer. J. Med. Sci.* **216**, 714.
10. Gilson, J. C., and Hugh-Jones, P. (1955). *Med. Res. Counc. Gt. Brit. Spec. Rep. Ser. 290.*
11. Rasmussen, D. "Papers and Proceedings of the National Conference on Medicine and the Federal Coal Mine Health and Safety Act of 1969," p. 139.
12. Lyon, J. P., Clarke, W. G., Hall, A. M., and Cotes, J. E. (1968). *Brit. Med. J.* **4**, 772.
12a. Macklein, P. J., and Mead, J. (1967). *J. Appl. Physiol.* **22**, 395.
13. Fletcher, C. M. (1948). *Brit. J. Prev. Soc. Med.* **1**, 1015.
14. Martin, J. E. (1954). *Amer. J. Pub. Health* **44**, 581.
15. Cochrane, A. L., Moore, F., and Thomas, J. (1961). *Tubercle* **42**, 64.
15a. Cochrane, A. L., and Higgins, I. T. T. (1961). *Brit. J. Prev. Soc. Med.* **15**, 1.
16. Levine, M. D., and Hunter, M. B. (1957). *J. Amer. Med. Ass.* **163**, 1.
17. Rogan, J. M., Chapman, P. J., Ashford, J. R., Duffield, D. P., Fay, J. W., and Rae, S. (1961). *Brit. Med. J.* **1**, 1337.

18. Higgins, I. T. T., Higgins, M. W., Lockshin, M. D., and Canale, N. (1968). *Brit. J. Ind. Med.* **25**, 165.
19. Higgins, I. T. T., Cochrane, A. L., Gilson, J. C., and Wood, C. H. (1959). *Brit. J. Ind. Med.* **16**, 255.
20. Higgins, I. T. T., and Cochrane, A. L. (1961). *Brit. J. Ind. Med.* **18**, 93.
21. Pemberton, J. (1956). *AMA Arch. Ind. Health* **13**, 529.
22. Waterman, D. H. (1957). *AMA Arch. Ind. Health* **15**, 447.
23. Medical Research Council Committee on Aetiology in Chronic Bronchitis (1969). *Lancet* **1**, 775.
24. American Thoracic Society, Committee on Diagnostic Standards for Non-Tuberculous Respiratory Diseases (1962). *Amer. Rev. Resp. Dis.* **85**, 762.
25. Higgins, I. T. T., Oldham, P. D., Cochrane, A. L., and Gilson, J. C. (1956). *Brit. Med. J.* **2**, 904.
26. Higgins, I. T. T., Gilson, J. C., Ferris, B. G., Waters, M. E., Campbell, H., and Higgins, M. W. (1968). *Amer. J. Pub. Health* **58**, 16, 67.
27. Rogan, J. (1970). *J. Occup. Med.* **12**, 321.
27a. Higgins, I. T. T., and Oldham, P. D. (1962). *Brit. J. Ind. Med.* **19**, 65.

5

General Pathology

John P. Wyatt

It has been said that the lung is a palimpsest (1), the writing on the lung papyrus being dependent on the impress of the legend, the quality of the ink, and the repetition of key characters in the inscription. Of greater importance is the value of the hermeneutics which can be extracted from the lung inscription, and the validity of this extracted translation is dependent on heuristic evidence from earlier writings and the maintained strength of the interpretation after critical study.

The historical interpretations of the "black ink" writings on the coal workers lung fabric were originally read in the first half of the nineteenth century. English and Scottish physicians (Pearson, Gregory, Marshall, Gibson, Thomson, Stratton, Jones) (2, 3) implicated fossilized carboniferous materials or "charcoal" of an exogenous nature as being responsible for pathological forms of "black lung" in coal miners. The autopsy descriptions and protocols of these soft-coal workers over a century ago actually present a narrative comparable to that documented for the mid-twentieth century coal worker: "the whole substance of the lungs was of a deep black color . . . and in the upper portions, they were of a solid or rubbery texture."

A few years later the problem ceased to be one of coal dust alone due to the recognition of permanent lung disease in other dusty trades and the growing attention in mining quarries to the presence of quartz-contaminated fields. On account of these findings, silicon dioxide was labeled the common and all-important fibrogenic inscriptive agent. This view persisted from the midnineteenth century until 1940, greatly

71

strengthened by Haldane's turn-of-the-century proclamation that coal dust held no dangers for life (3). Collis reechoed this pronouncement by adding that "miner's asthma" had disappeared; its cause and nature were of no further concern (3). Progressive pulmonary disabilities in coal workers were attributed exclusively to the sclerosing powers of rock dust until Gough (4) in 1940 demonstrated that in workers in the holds of ships, shovelling coal (which was relatively free of silica), developed a distinctive and separable form of pneumoconiosis. After a massive survey of coal miners in South Wales, Hart and Aslett supported this discovery by the documentation of an identical pneumoconiosis in that coal mining group. Since that time numerous investigators have been analyzing the diverse ramifications of the natural history of coal workers' pneumoconiosis (5, 6).

ANATOMY OF THE DISTAL RESPIRATORY UNIT

For a basic understanding of the coal pigment lesion and the morphogenic pathways that determine the progress of the pathologic condition after the initial establishment of the lesion, one must refer back to the anatomy of normal aerating tissue.

Our major concern is with the terminal respiratory bronchiole. This is the fundamental site for the deposition of dust, but of greater importance is that the anatomic placement of the respiratory bronchioles predetermines much of the rationale for our current morphological classification of obstructive airway disease (7).

The terminal respiratory bronchioles, usually a half-dozen in number, are more or less centrally located within the secondary lobule. The secondary lobule is composed of approximately three or four dozen primary lobules derived from dividing respiratory bronchioles. The peripheral definity of the secondary lobule is due to the extensions and enclosures of connective tissue, which are in continuity with the lung hilar tissue. This peripheral envelope of connective tissue, originally described by Miller (8), is best illustrated in inflated, fixed, and transected specimens of whole lung. The connective tissue envelope is more easily recognized in the upper half of the lung and with less ease in its lower third. In this respect, the upper half of the human lung, on the basis of comparative anatomy, is like the compartmented lobular lung of the cow, whereas the lower third, where secondary lobule septation is poor, is akin to the noncompartmented, "facile collateral drift" lung of the dog. This sharper definition of the secondary lobule by peripheral connective tissue may explain the much greater frequency of bullous fields in the upper half of the lung in contrast with their rarity in the lower pulmonary regions. Under the aerotraumatic effects of obstructive airway disease, the connective tissue mantle is most resistant: a bulla is a completely destroyed secondary lobule with retention of its peripheral envelope of connective tissue. A bullous region is composed of multiples of destroyed lobules.

The centrally situated respiratory bronchioles have three orders of size, progressively decreasing, until the respiratory bronchiole of the third order gives rise, in an anatomically repetitive dichotomous fashion, to air ducts. These air ducts, of a luminal caliber approximately equivalent to the respiratory bronchiole of the third order, give origin to their penultimate derivatives—the air sacs. The term *respiratory bronchiole* distinguishes these structures from the terminal bronchiole, and the use of the term *respiratory* indicates that a single primary generation of air sacs buds off the respiratory bronchiole. Oxygen can diffuse directly into lobular units of different bronchiolar origin but closely apposed anatomically aerating tissue. The air ducts bud off directly into "geometrically" arranged air sacs, analogous in a fashion to stalls opening from a main corridor.

The microanatomic location of the centrally placed respiratory bronchioles is, from a functional sense, a strategic one (9). The respiratory bronchioles are the direct channels which divide up into air ducts and control the flow of fresh air into a significant functional gas exchange terrain. Of equal importance in this gas exchange aerating field is the vascular structure that distributes low-pressure pulmonary arterial blood into it. The lobular arteriole has an intimate association with its companion, the respiratory bronchiole, until it divides up into the omnidirectional capillary bed at the level of the first orders of the respiratory bronchiole. Although not of major significance under normal conditions, it is at this level that bronchial artery flow contributions can be demonstrated.

The identification of the lobular arteriole is facilitated by the postmortem filling of these vessels by latex. The use of latex which can be sectioned by conventional methods reinforces the anatomic concept that essential structures are easily identified in health and disease, particularly after special preparation. The use of such media enhances the functional interpretations of the distal respiratory unit.

After traversing the terrain of the defined aerating unit related to the lobular arteriole, the oxygenated blood enters into venules, and these are gathered together within the peripheral connective tissues of Miller as the pulmonary venous blood destined for the left heart. Perivenous lymphatics accompany the veins in the connective tissue which defines the secondary lobule.

THE MORBID ANATOMY OF COAL WORKERS' LUNG

In general, two distinctive gross patterns of lung alteration in the coal worker are readily recognized (10).

In the lungs of coal miners with only a few years of exposure, and

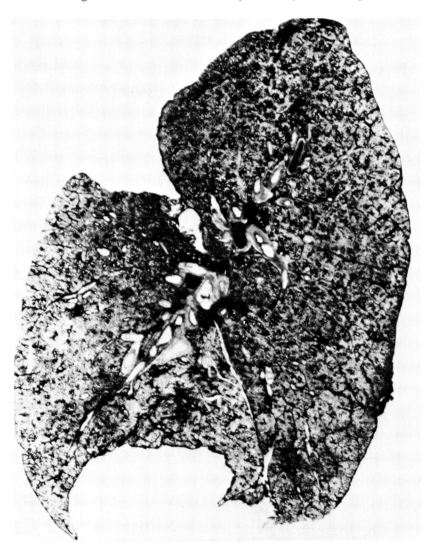

FIG. 1. Lung: Simple pneumoconiosis. Extensive distribution of coal pigment uniformly throughout the lung. Greatest concentration of dust in upper regions. Whole lung macrosection. ×0.25.

apparently associated with little ventilatory impairment, the outstanding feature of the autopsied lung is its color (Fig. 1). The lungs are generally gray-black in color, with the pigmentary changes bilateral and symmetrical in distribution. In the conventional transection of the lung, minute discrete nodules, approximately 1–4 mm in size, roll under the fingers on palpation, but they are difficult to visualize unless the lung has been inflated. The pleural surfaces reflect the general black discoloration since frequently the coal pigment creates black lines which outline the triangular or trapezoidal patterns of the secondary lobules. This blue-black veining is reminiscent of Roquefort cheese.

The other and often the end response in advanced CWP is the presence of rounded masses of dense black tissue. A few of the massive nodules are usually found in the upper half of the lung and have fissures or cracks in the rubbery scar. These fissures leak inky black fluid on gross sectioning. (It was possible to write on the back of the giant paper sections of the lungs prepared for whole lung sectioning with this "ink" originally collected at the time of blocking.) This form of CWP is spoken of as progressive massive fibrosis (PMF). It causes a severe respiratory disability and has frequently resulted in premature death. With the attainment of a certain degree of simple pneumoconiosis, it appears that this fibrosing pulmonary condition can also be found in miners who had left their occupation a few years before.

The hilar lymph nodes in both early and end responses are enlarged, have an intense black color, and show diffuse bands of scar tissue radiating throughout medulla and cortex. Littoral cell proliferation and agminates of dust macrophages are conspicuous.

Owing to the limited amount of autopsied material, either personally obtained or submitted for whole lung assessment, only the general epidemiologic trend can be commented on. The incidence of simple pneumoconiosis and the subsequent development of massive fibrosis appear to bear a direct relationship to the years of exposure and bulk mass of dust; the particular type of underground employment appears to be of less importance since all soft-coal workers possessed the characteristic macular lesion.

Anatomic Distribution of Coal-Mined Dust

After a few years of exposure the coal-mined dust reveals an extensive, diffuse, and remarkably uniform distribution throughout the secondary lobules of the whole lung (Figs. 1 and 2). Examination of whole lung sections of miners who had the longer periods of employment underground reveals a greater concentration of dust in the upper region of the lung. The dust accumulates in and around the all-important respiratory bron-

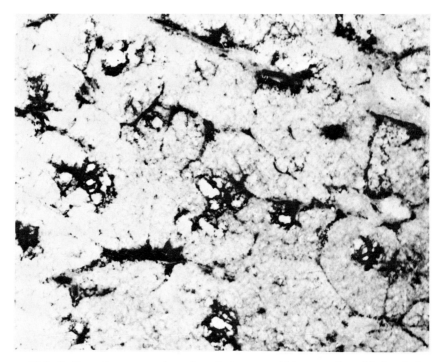

FIG. 2. Central concentration of coal pigment within secondary lobule. A few foci show bronchiolar dilatation. Most of the secondary lobules outlined by connective tissue are lightly pigmented. Secondary lobules have triangular, quadrilateral, or hexagonal cross section patterns. Sector from whole lung paper section. ×9.2.

chiole, particularly in the proximal orders. The concentration of the dust in these bronchioles and at their bifurcational or postdivisional points implies a relationship between flow of particle, dust size, and "fall out" points of the dust in these air conductive pathways. In essence, the initial inceptive and crucial lesion in coal workers' pneumoconiosis is a mantle of macrophages burdened with coal-mined dust enmeshed in fibrous tissue around the respiratory bronchiole and lobular arteriole (11).

Early Macular "Emphysema"

Although the initial lesion is one of coal pigmentation, there is almost from the beginning in this type of pneumoconiosis the constant companion of bronchiolar dilatation (Fig. 3). This early dilatation was labeled originally "focal emphysema" by pathologists studying autopsy material from miners of the Rhonda Fach in South Wales. Considerable controversy has resulted from the use of this particular term; one is the concern

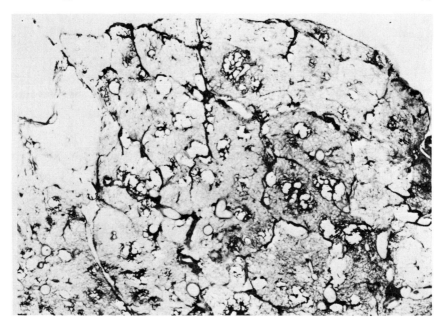

FIG. 3. Twelve or more secondary lobules outlined by pigment deposition in the peripheral mantles of connective tissue which demarcate these macroanatomical lobules. Pigmentary foci and respiratory bronchiolar air pools centrally situated. Sector of whole lung paper section. ×8.2.

of the clinicians on the lack of correlation with physiologic function; the other is the confinement of the term to mean only dilatation of the terminal air conducting pathways. A major gain has been a morphological one. With the recognition of the central lobular demarcation of the coal workers' lesion (Fig. 4), the other forms of nonindustrial emphysema are oriented now around a universally accepted anatomical classification based on the secondary lobule (7).

In the conventional histologic preparation (Fig. 5), the coal macule presents a characteristic pattern. The stellate pigment freckle, with the air pools between the radiating "spokes" of the pigmentary lesion, extends down in the form of irregular tails of pigmentation deposited in the distal orders of respiratory bronchioles. The lessening concentrations and irregularities in coal deposition are determined by the microanatomy. This anatomical gradient of coal dust and the absence of a fibrosing response, in addition to the easy acceptance of authoritative statements in the past that coal dust was inert, may explain the oversight of the key lesion in earlier pathologic studies of the coal miners lung.

By serial reconstructions, the exact location of the carboniferous pigment deposition can be determined. The profile of pigment deposition in

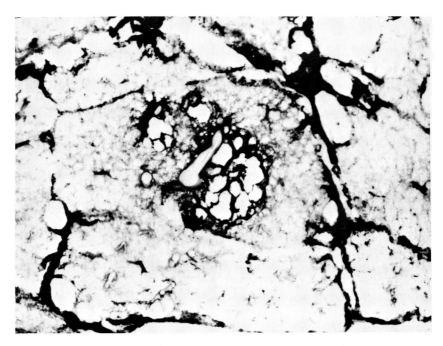

FIG. 4. Close up of secondary lobule from Fig. 3. The centrally situated lobular arteriole, filled with latex, is enmeshed in the confluent air pools outlined by coal pigment. Paralobular veins and lymphatics are at periphery of secondary lobule. Sector of whole lung paper section. ×12.

the respiratory bronchiole of the Appalachian coal miner is identical to that demonstrated by Heppleston for the South Wales coal miner (12). The pigment lines the walls of all three orders of the respiratory bronchiole, but to a lesser degree in the bronchiolar third order and air ducts. Free dust particles are demonstrable in the sacs arising from the primary air duct. The greatest concentration of dust is either intramural or outside the outer borders of the bronchioles; this pigment pattern is responsible for the "spokes" of the lesion [Figs. 6(a)–6(d)]. The dust lesion in simple pneumoconiosis is, in essence, a predominance of dust and a minimal fibrosing response.

In the stereoscopic viewing of well-formed macules there is an intense accumulation of coal; *a fortiorari* is the recognition of early breaches or dissolutions in the wall of the respiratory bronchioles. In manipulations of the macule under the stereoscope and in submerged specimens, the formed coal lesion has a distinct tension of its own and moves as a total "stiffened" unit within its own confluent air pool. Our stiffened form under the stereoscope probably is the same as Heppleston's "retrogressive

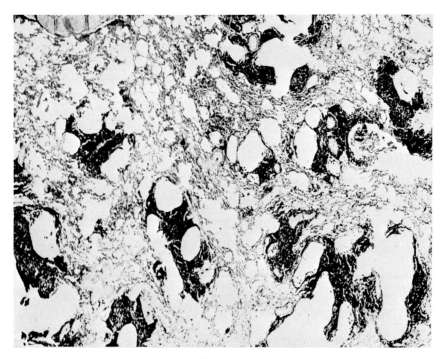

FIG. 5. The conventional view of "anthracosis" which demonstrates uniform concentrations of coal pigment delineating dilated spaces due to ec⁺asia of respiratory bronchioles. Lung; hematoxylin and eosin. ×60.

and cicatrized" histologic macule which morphogenically followed his earlier "formative and proliferative" macule (12).

The pathogenesis of the bronchiolar dilatation (South Wales "focal" emphysema) and its later mural dissolution is unknown. Heppleston contended that the coal dust per se is the causa causans of the focal emphysema. The coal dust burden influences the lung mechanically; eventually the tissue contractile elements of the lung atrophies, and irreversible emphysematous changes develope. Another explanation for the emphysema may be that the progressive silting up of the distal respiratory unit leads to dissolution of the cellular packs of burdened macrophages, and their lysosomal enzymes, liberated by cell disintegration, progressively destroy the supporting tissue of the airways.

The Coal Pigment–Vascular Lesion

A lesion of importance, which was not stressed in the earlier studies of CWP in South Wales colliers, is the anatomic association of the dust

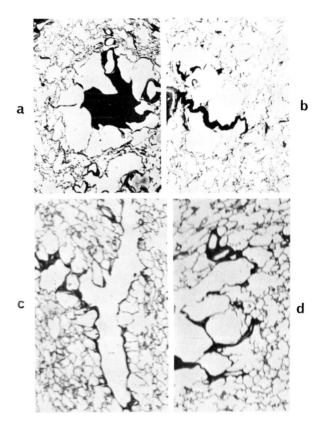

FIG. 6. Four views reflecting the concentration and petering out of coal pigment in relationship to the microanatomy of the dividing respiratory bronchiole: (a) macule with companion emphysema; (b) pigmentary tail at second-order of respiratory bronchiole; (c) progressive disappearance of pigment as bronchiole divides into air ducts; (d) pigment present in bronchiolar air duct walls. Lung; hematoxylin and eosin. ×45.

with the respiratory bronchiole, together with its obvious relationship to the apposed lobular arteriole.

The coal-dust-laden cells penetrate through the outer walls of the respiratory bronchioles and outside smooth muscle and are deposited on the adventitial wall of the juxtaposed lobular arterioles (Fig. 7). Histologic sectioning reveals coal pigment between the bundles of smooth muscle of the arteriolar wall. Progressive accumulations thicken up the anatomical interstitial tissue between the bronchiolar wall and vascular adventitia; in advanced focal lesions, an impression of vascular narrowing is gained by stereoscopic viewing.

As a later phenomenon, the pulmonary capillaries at the peripheral

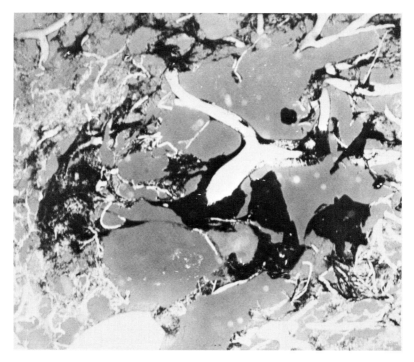

FIG. 7. A "stereoscopic" view of a coal macule in which the associated lobular arteriole has been previously injected with latex (white). Early dissolution of respiratory bronchiolar wall and associated capillary bed are demonstrated. Sector of inflated, formalin fixed lung block. ×60.

attentuated portions of the macular unit are broken up, and the central portion of the lobular bed is absent (Fig. 7). With further progression of the dissolutive emphysematous process, the labyrinthinal or omnidirectional capillary bed is found to be destroyed by the fenestrations and breaches in the related aerating tissue. There is a genuine reduction in the microvascular bed, and the residue of blood pathways is unidirectional and forms part of the connective tissue covering derived from peripheral remnants of the lobule.

This circumferential dust yoke around the pulmonary arteriole bed forces the question which was originally framed by physiologic studies (13): What is the possible role of the constrictive pigment yoke around the lobular arteriole in the reduction of oxygen transfer in CWP? With progressive coal dust accumulations and other related changes, a dual impediment to delivery of blood and fresh air may develop. The impediment may be unequally distributed between ventilatory and perfusional channels; the cidevant emphasis upon ventilatory studies may have initially cast into umbrage this potential perfusional derangement which is anatomically related to dust accumulations. Although the morphologic model of nonindustrial centrilobular emphysema was an acceptable scaffold in explaining functional mismatching between ventilation and perfusion (14) at a secondary lobular level, a similar morphologic template has not yet been found to give clinical and physiological support to the centrilobular pigmentary emphysematous lesion.

Progression of Pulmonary Emphysema

Of the lungs from autopsied miners who have worked in southern Illinois coal fields, Kentucky mining communities, and Virginia coal fields, a few show progression of the emphysematous component (Fig. 8). The progression of the emphysema in the few available examples show the extension of the dissolutive process from the centrilobular zones of the secondary lobule until the major portion of the lobule disappears.

The term progression, as used here, means the morphologic advance-

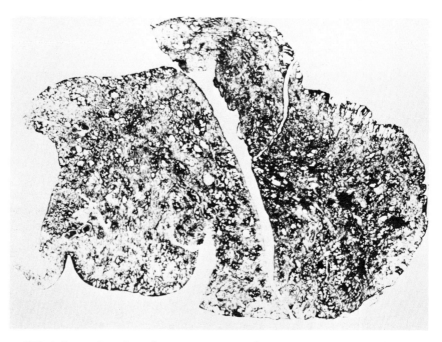

FIG. 8. Lung: Complicated pneumoconiosis. Pulmonary emphysema in coal worker, with lung distention and dissolution broadly distributed, with peripheral areas showing greatest destruction. Several black nodules of progressive fibrosis noted in upper half of lung. Whole lung paper macrosection. ×0.2.

ment of the condition throughout the entire lobe, largely achieved through continuing fusion of mural fenestrations until there is a complete disappearance of identifiable or oriented anatomical structures. The use of the term progression does not mean that the responsible pathogenetic mechanism has been established.

The lobule is often damaged in an eccentric fashion, and this spatial irregularity persists in the evolution of the emphysematous process from the small to the much larger confluent air pools (Fig. 9). These larger emphysematous areas are often delimited by a coal-black rim of tissue, partially composed of remnants of bronchiolar walls and partially of connective tissue concurrently tattooed with pigment. The "progressive extension of the related focal emphysema over even wider areas of lung tissue" has been commented on by other investigators (11, 12).

In whole lung sections prepared from an advanced case of CWP, the emphysema is more obvious at the lung periphery, but the centrilobular foci of emphysema remains uniformly distributed throughout the lung. In this respect, the emphysema of CWP is not a repetition of nonindustrial centrilobular emphysema. In this latter type of morphologic emphysema the greatest degrees of the lung dissolution are seen in the upper

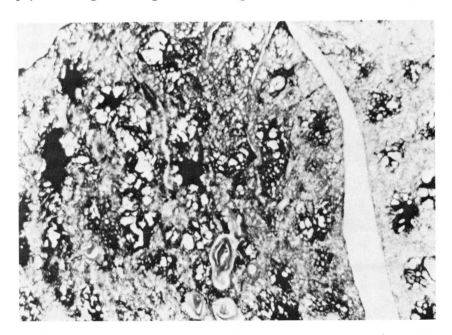

FIG. 9. Heavy coal burden in lung with some of the macular emphysematous regions showing early appositional confluence to give irregularities in pattern of emphysema. Sector of whole lung paper macrosection. ×8.3.

third and posterior portions of the lung with much less lung destruction in the lower pulmonary regions. In a few examples of coal miners lung, diffuse panlobular emphysema is observed, with the coal pigment entrapped at an air sac level. The evidence of the key centrilobular coal macule is difficult to discern, although lengthy periods of exposure to coal dust are clinically documented in these miners (Figs. 10–12). The macular pattern is often overshadowed by the extent of emphysema, but on viewing multiple whole lung paper sections, discrete and characteristic macular units are still recognizable; the characterization of the pattern is often difficult, particularly in ex-coal miners whose employment had been years earlier.

In those instances of extensive emphysema with a sparse population of coal macules, the two lung dissolutive processes are probably not causally related. A recent survey of coal workers' emphysema by quantitative methods indicates that the pulmonary ventilatory impairment due to the emphysematous component has a greater correlation with finer dust changes than in those miners with coarser changes (15). It has also been commented on that miners with negative chest radiographs may have considerable pulmonary disability. These paradoxes between morphology and pulmonary function have produced a lively but pertinent medical correspondence (16, 17).

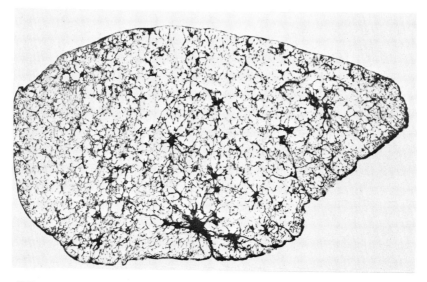

FIG. 10. Lung: Complicated pneumoconiosis. A lobe of a grossly emphysematous lung, in which the background of the pattern is centrilobular in form. A few irregular nodules of progressive fibrosis are scattered throughout the lung. Whole lung paper macrosection. ×0.3.

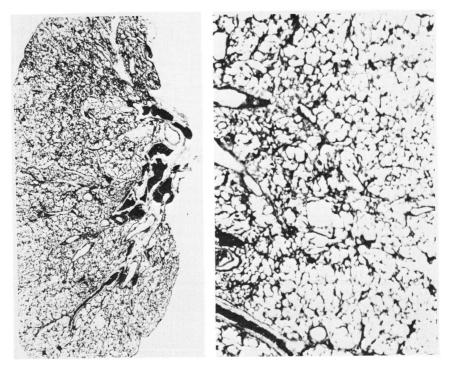

FIG. 11. Two views: (left) whole lung paper section (×0.2) showing diffuse form of panlobular emphysema and intensely black hilar lymph nodes; (right) sector view (×6) of same lung in a coal miner showing extensive emphysema and diffuse filigreed pigment pattern through lobular tissue.

Despite the difficulties of analyzing histologic chronic bronchitis on a whole lung basis, this group of miners with noticeable emphysema represents a sampling in which quantitative methods directed not only at the emphysema but also at the conducting airways might close this hiatus in the natural history of bronchitis–emphysema in coal workers. Although the epithelial field response of hypertrophy and hyperplasia, particularly of mucous gland and goblet cell, is a morphologic indicator of chronic bronchitis, it should be remembered that it is also a common response to a polygon of irritative agents.

In general, the association of generalized emphysema is not to be equated with the degree of fibrosis. This lack of association is also a feature of nonindustrial centrilobular emphysema. From the whole lung view of both groups, a reemphasis of the relationship of bronchitis to pulmonary emphysema is pivotal to future investigations into pulmonary disease in coal workers.

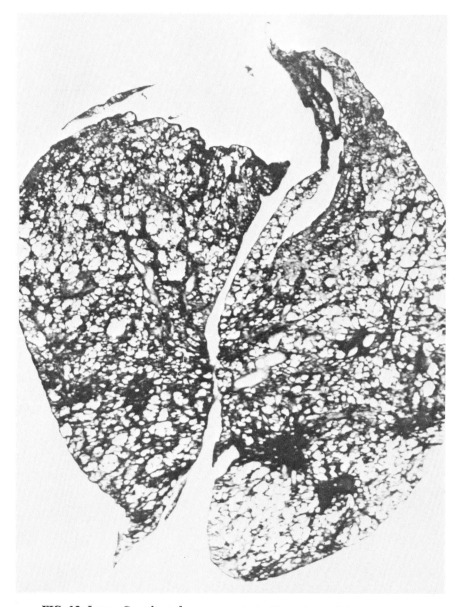

FIG. 12. Lung: Complicated pneumoconiosis. Extensive nodular progressive massive fibrosis and widespread advanced emphysema. Whole lung paper macrosection. ×0.25.

Evolution of the Fibrotic Component

With the continuing increase in the dust burden over the years, a significant proportion of the miners have developed another distinctive tissue alteration. A fibrosing response emerges, first on an individual nodular basis and later by an autochthonous progression. These pulmonary scar manifestations are labeled as progressive massive fibrosis (Fig. 13). These fibrotic nodules are often concentric in shape, but with advancement in degree and extent, polymorphic patterns are observed. The nodules show a gradual increment in size from 0.5 cm in diameter up to 3–4 cm or even larger or the fibrosing response is present as broad irregular scars. This massive fibrosis is found usually in the upper portion of the lung. The nodular foci are jet black in color, and retained within the interwoven fibrous tissue are large agminations of coal and mixed pigment. From the standpoint of progression, the early reticular fibrosis (Masson trichrome green) which was demonstrated in the "stiff" macules

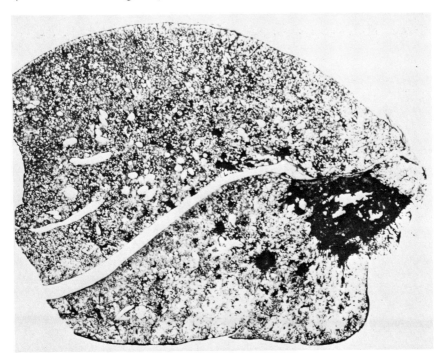

FIG. 13. Lung: Complicated pneumoconiosis. The dominant alteration is that of progressive massive fibrosis in the upper portions of the lung. A few black satellite nodules of varying dimensions are separated from the larger cavitary form of massive fibrosis. Whole lung paper macrosection. ×0.4.

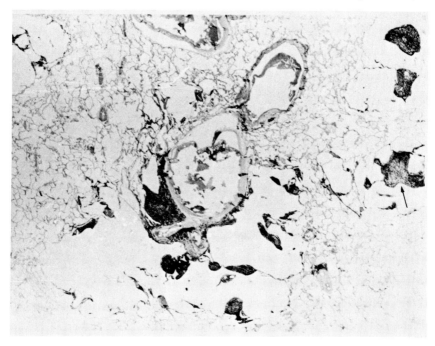

FIG. 14. A number of macular lesions with several showing early collagenic fibrosis (arrow). The close anatomic relationship between bronchiole and arteriole is revealed. The "spokes" of the macule show knobs of dust cells and thin strands of collagen. Lung; hematoxylin and eosin. ×46.

(lifted out by stereoscopic manipulations) is, in contracted macules, replaced by an isomorphic scar radiating out from the macular center. The fibrosis is minimal, but if there is a pattern of distribution to the fibrosis it is radial in direction and totally unlike that due to quartz (Fig. 14). The concentric redundant fibrosis, so characteristic of injury due to silica, is not found at any stage in the developing macules in our postmortem material.

After microincineration, performed at different temperature readings or following acid treatment, birefringent particles are sparsely distributed in our polarizing light studies. The birefringent particles remaining after microincineration are scattered haphazardly throughout the polymorphic nodules. It is only in the early "isomorphic" scars that a directional orientation to the birefringent crystals is noted. The Belt phenomenon (1) (peripheral mantling of the silica nodule by polarizing crystals) is not observed in the macules subjected to this type of technologic examination. Spatial distribution of refractile particles is probably of greater significance than dependence on visual assessment since old silica particles lose their birefringency and silicates may be doubly refractile. Chemical determinations for free silica are always extremely low in these macules (10).

The pulmonary disability portrait of progressive massive fibrosis has been stressed by clinical investigators in some of the United States coal fields, but there is a task for pathologists to undertake an integrative study on the autopsied lungs in these patients, particularly in view of the fact that the emergence of PMF out of the large potential pool of simple pneumoconioses appears to vary between different mining communities. In our series, progressive massive fibrosis is not a common feature, but this is probably due to the limitation in numbers within our original group. From this group of cases, no comparison as to the frequency of PMF can be drawn, although three geographically distinct regions— southern Illinois, West Virginia, and Kentucky—were sampled. All three areas had examples of PMF.

One feature in our whole lung study of fibrosis in CWP is the absence of morphologic evidence to consider that fusion or coalescence of nodular lesions is responsible for PMF. Furthermore, in previous whole lung studies from workers dying from pure or mixed silicosis, there are three features of restrictive lung disease (18) that are not observed in CWP. In silicosis, (i) the respiratory bronchioles are narrowed; (ii) in association with the concentric nodules of silicosis there is evidence of tractional influences upon surrounding aerating tissue; and (iii) the larger masses in silicosis frequently reveal that their massive size is due to the binding together of initially discrete micronodular tissue (18).

The morphogenic pathways that integrate punctiform nodular and progressive massive fibrosis have not been defined. The transient phases between the reticular nodule (Fig. 14) and the massive fibrotic lesion await further elucidation, not only from the standpoint of quantitative dust content at the individual scar level, but by a search for other putative factors possibly concerned in CWP collagen production.

Speculation on the causation of the progressive fibrosis and centrinodular necrosis in the massive scars indicates a wide divergence of views. Anatomic parameters frequently are recalled to explain progressive fibrosis on an infectional basis, particularly in the case of tuberculosis. The relatively low recovery of tubercle bacilli from the fibronecrotic areas (30–40%) enhances the value of (a) the predilection of the massive scars for upper lobes which is common to both pathologic conditions, CWP, and fibrocaseous tuberculosis; and (b) the association of lymphomononuclear cells with hyalinized scar, as morphologic support for the postulate of an infectious origin for PMF. Belt also subscribes to the infectional genesis of PMF by the coinage of the word *koniophthisis* for the progressive cicatrizing lesion.

A second conjecture on the fibronecrotic nature of PMF stresses the fact that microvascular compromization sustains local tissue hypoxia which in turn provokes hyalin fibrosis. On a more extensive basis small vessel bed obliteration produces frank infarction and cavitation of tissue.

A third premise as to the etiology of nodular fibrosis in coal pneumoconiosis proffers the findings that the nodule formation from its inception to the ultimate development of delimited necrosis represents an immunobiologic process which may operate, particularly in those hypersensitive miners who possess a circulating rheumatoid factor (Caplan's syndrome) (19).

As indicated earlier, the two pathologic processes of fibrosis and emphysema have been found together in a number of examples of PMF (Fig. 13). It is apparent that the fibrotic component is not specifically oriented to the anatomic pattern of the emphysema. The inference from this morphologic observation is that the fibrosing elements do not act in a mechanical or physical manner in the production of the pulmonary emphysema.

MORPHOLOGIC "COR PULMONALE" IN CWP

Evidence from clinical, physiologic and integrated pathologic studies indicates that the most important factor leading to the development of pulmonary hypertension is chronic hypoxia (20). With persistence of chronic hypoxia, pulmonary hypertension becomes a cardinal feature of chronic respiratory disease. There is a contemporary need for accurate and reproducible analyses in different lung investigative centers charged with responsibility of investigating coal workers' pneumoconiosis.

The adaptive cardiac response of right ventricular hypertrophy measured by quantitative methods in concordance with similar mensural techniques applied to the pulmonic aerating and blood distributional beds (7, 21) is essential, particularly in those clinical patients who have had physiologic performance studies over a period of years.

Simple pneumoconiosis rarely causes right ventricular hypertrophy, but a recent study in Australia suggests that with increasing grades of coal pneumoconiosis there are progressive increments in right ventricle thickness (22). Hypertrophy of the right ventricle (greater than 72 g in weight and most myocardial fibres measuring greater than 12 μ in diameter) is not a prominent feature in the majority of our examples of

CWP. The limited sample of CWP in our series and the paucity of cases in which quantitative measures of the pulmonary and cardiac tissues is possible may account for this difference. The general trend of the relationship is that those cases with hypertrophy of the right chamber have the greatest degree of fibrosis and emphysema. In this respect, genuine cases of CWP with centrilobular macular lesions do not show the heightened incidence of right-sided cardiac hypertrophy that has been recorded with limited degrees of nonindustrial centrilobular emphysema (20). With the superimposition of bronchitis as well as a compromised vascular bed produced by the PMF, pulmonary hypertension is apparently greatly augmented, and right ventricular hypertrophy is found to be extremely common (23).

CONCLUSION

Although many aspects of the natural history of coal workers' pneumoconiosis have been carefully delineated, numerous gaps in our knowledge of this pulmonary disability remain.

Many of these hiatuses exist in correlative relationships between physiologic surveys and morphologic answers. There is a need to establish (i) an adequate explanation for defects in oxygen transfer in the earlier phases of some of the patients suffering from coal workers' pneumoconiosis; (ii) the factor(s) responsible for the emergence of progressive massive fibrosis in limited numbers out of a large active pool of miners with uncomplicated pneumoconiosis; (iii) information on the micro- and macroenvironmental or genetic differences in miners that are responsible for the augmented emphysematous lung dissolution in some miners who have limited coal burdens within their lungs; and (iv) a precise anatomic assessment of the adaptive cardiac changes to more clearly reflect the progression of the pulmonary disease complex.

Albeit the suppression of dust in coal mining areas may curtail the number of new cases of coal workers' pneumoconiosis which develope, there is an impress upon the medical profession for more sophisticated probings to mark out the vulnerable respiratory system and the subtle or deviant forms of lung injury which may be presently submerged under the contemporary crude portrait of the distinctive pulmonary disability shared by so many of today's coal miners.

REFERENCES

1. Belt, T., and Ferris, A. A. (1942). *Med. Res. Counc. Gt. Brit. Spec. Rep. Ser.* 243, 203.

2. Cummins, S. L., and Sladden, A. F. (1930). *J. Pathol. Bacteriol.* **33**, 1095.

3. Fletcher, C. W. (1948). *Brit. Med. J.* **1**, 1015.

4. Gough, J. (1940). *J. Pathol. Bacteriol.* **51**, 277.

5. Gibson, J. C., and Hugh-Jones, P. (1955). *Med. Res. Counc. Gt. Brit. Spec. Rep. Ser.* **290**, 1.

6. Rae, S. (1971). *Brit. Med. Bull.* **27**, 53.

7. Fischer, V. W., Sweet, A. C., and Wyatt, J. P. (1964). *Amer. Rev. Resp. Dis.* **89**, 533.

8. Miller, W. S. (1950). *In* "The Lung," 2nd ed. Thomas, Springfield, Ill.

9. Adamson, I. Y. R., Bowden, D. H., and Wyatt, J. P. (1968). *Arch. Pathol.* **86**, 671.

10. Wyatt, J. P. (1960). *Arch. Ind. Health* **21**, 445.

11. Heppleston, A. G. (1947). *J. Pathol. Bacteriol.* **49**, 453.

12. Heppleston, A. G. (1954). *J. Pathol. Bacteriol.* **64**, 51.

13. Rasmussen, D. L. (1970). *In* "Papers and Proceedings of the National Conference on Medicine and the Federal Coal Mine Health and Safety Act of 1969," pp. 139–147. Div. Environ. Health Sci., Univ. Calif., Howard Univ.

14. Bowden, D. H., and Wyatt, J. P. (1970). *Pathol. Annu.* pp. 279–307.

15. Campbell, H., Gough, J., Lyons, J. P., and Ryder, R. (1970). *Brit. Med. J.* **3**, 481.

16. Gibson, J. C., and Oldbeam, P. D. (1970). *Brit. Med. J.* **3**, 305.

17. Jacobsen, M., Muir, D. C. F., and Rae, S. (1970). *Brit. Med. J.* **3**, 305.

18. Ishikawa, S., and Wyatt, J. P. (1970). *Hum. Pathol.* **1**, 289.

19. Caplan, A., Payne, R. B., and Withey, J. L. (1962). *Thorax* **17**, 205.

20. Ishikawa, S., and Wyatt, J. P. (1968). *In* "Form and Function in the Human Lung" (G. Cumming and L. B. Hunt, eds.), pp. 170–181. Livingstone, Edinburgh and London.

21. Butler, C., and Kleinerman, J. (1970). *Am. Rev. Resp. Dis.* **102**, 886.

22. McKenzie, H. I., Outhred, K. G., and White, K. H. (1970). *Med. J. Aust.* **1**, 950.

23. Naeye, R. L. (1970). *Amer. Assoc. Pathol. Bacteriol.,* Annual Meeting (Abstr.).

6

Structural Features in Appalachian Coal Workers

Richard L. Naeye

In recent years coal workers' pneumoconiosis has been widely accepted as a disease entity, but there remain uncertainties about its prevalence, severity, and pathogenesis. In a survey of published Appalachian roentgenographic studies, Morgan found a prevalence of pneumoconiosis ranging from 10–55% in soft-coal workers and from 30–76% in anthracite workers (1). It is difficult to interpret these observations, because correlations are often poor between such roentgenographic findings, symptoms, physical findings, and physiologic abnormalities (2, 3). Even the pulmonary structural abnormalities responsible for CWP have not been completely defined, especially since they vary from one region to another. It is also unclear what the proportionate contributions of coal dust, other mine dusts and fumes, and smoking and community air contaminants might be to the development of CWP.

More comprehensive European studies have only partial relevance to the disorder in the United States because of probable differences in prevalence and severity of CWP between the two continents. Prior to 1970, dust levels in many western European mines were lower than in most United States mines. Comparisons are further complicated by the fact that the disease process may vary in severity not only within national boundaries, but also from area to area in a single coal seam. To resolve some of these uncertainties a quantitative, morphologic study was undertaken of lung and heart structure on 322 representative United States Appalachian coal miners.

Case Selection

The first group of 322 miners studied was subdivided on the basis of rank of coal mined (4, 5). Many reports have suggested that the higher the rank of coal, the greater the prevalence of pulmonary disease (1, 5). In the ranking system, the higher-ranked coals contain the most fixed carbon, have the greatest caloric value, and have the least volatile matter (6). The coals mined in Appalachia have a wide range of ranks, but fortunately for those who study CWP, the coal mined in any small geographic area is usually rather uniform in rank so that local workers have usually been exposed to only one type of coal. The first group of 113 miners had always mined low-rank, high-volatile bituminous coal in three counties of southwestern Pennsylvania or in a nearby county in West Virginia (4, 5). In this area the coal seams are quite high, often about 6 ft. The second group of 58 men had always mined higher-rank, low-volatile bituminous coal in Cambria and Somerset counties of central Pennsylvania. At many points, coal seams in this area are lower in height than the seams in southwestern Pennsylvania. The third group of 141 men had always mined high-rank anthracite coal in Schuylkill, Luzerne, and Carbon counties of eastern Pennsylvania (5).

The free silica content of coal dust is low, seldom greater than 3%, in all of the aforementioned areas. However, such measurements do not always reflect the actual exposure of the men to silica. The mine dust concentration of free silica is sometimes high for certain workers, such as electric locomotive operators and roof bolters who encounter pulverized sand or drill into silica bearing rock. Actual rock structure also has an influence on silica exposure. The bituminous seams are usually horizontal or have low grades, often minimizing the exposure to pulverized sand used for traction. Where the seams are continuously high, there may be little need to remove intervening silica bearing rock. In contrast, the anthracite seams are usually sharply inclined, often making it necessary to remove intervening hard rock.

The cases selected were located through a search of autopsy files by the author who visited each hospital and read every autopsy protocol which involved a male over 20 years of age who died between 1960 and 1968 (4, 5, 7). Cases were considered for selection when the autopsy protocol mentioned excessive pigment, parenchymal nodules, fibrosis, or a history of mining. Occupational and clinical information was extracted from clinical charts. Cases were included in the study only after occupational exposure underground had been confirmed by a responsible relative. The following information was obtained: (a) number of years in each underground mine, with dates, (b) specific jobs in each mine, (c) nonmining jobs, with dates, (d) if retired, date when quit mining, and (4) smoking history. These family contacts disclosed 32 miners who never smoked, 24 who smoked pipe or cigars, and 88 who smoked cigarettes (7). Men were classified as smokers only when the habit had extended most of their adult lives. The cigarette smokers were subclassified on the basis of their consumption in late years.

The method of case finding had some inherent limitations (4). Autopsies are rare on younger miners who die, so that most men included in the study were both old and retired. Mean age for the various groups ranged from 65 to 68 years and underground exposure to coal dust to more than 30 years. Most men worked through the period when the mines were being mechanized, so they had been exposed to dust generated by a variety of mining methods. Attempts were made to make case selection representative of miners dying in each geographic area by using only cases from general hospitals; cases from hospitals or clinics specializing in pulmonary diseases were excluded.

A serial section study of lung tissue was undertaken on a fourth group of 10 bituminous miners, selected because they had many small pulmonary arteries with no abnormal intimal or medial tissue elements (8). The absence of such abnormalities made possible a quantitative analysis of the vessels' medial muscle.

Methods

Methods used in the study have been reported previously (4, 5, 7, 8). Quantitative, histologic studies were undertaken on individual cases without prior knowledge of age, type of coal, smoking history, gross cardiac, or pulmonary findings.

Dust Macules and Nodules. Macules of coal dust are the primary lesions in coal workers' pneumoconiosis (4, 9). The percent of lung comprised of such macules and larger fibrotic nodules was measured by the microscopic technique of Dunnill (10). With this technique, multiple randomly selected microscopic sections are subjected to microscopic point counting. Four to twelve tissue blocks from each case were cut at 5 μ and duplicate sections were stained with hematoxylin and eosin and Verhoeff's and Van Gieson's stains. Ten randomly selected fields in each section were carefully observed and each superimposed point categorized as to (a) dust macule or fibrotic nodule and (b) other tissue or space. The number of macule or nodule divided by the total number of points counted gives the percent of lung comprised of macules and nodules.

Silica Content of Macules and Nodules. An attempt was made to quantitate indirectly the silica content of dust macules and nodules by counting points of polarized light within a grid superimposed on the macules and nodules (4). Values were recorded in points of light per 10,000 μ^2. Microincineration at 600°C followed by concentrated hydrochloric acid for 30 minutes reduced the count by about 50%, indicating that at least half of the points were silica crystals (4).

Collagen Content of Macules and Nodules. Duplicate sections of lung were stained with (a) Verhoeff's and Van Gieson's and (b) trichrome stains to demonstrate collagen. Collagen content of each macule and nodule in a case was visually graded on a scale of 1+ to 4+, and then a mean value was determined for the case and for various groupings of miners. The grades were as follows: 0, no visible collagen; 1+, thin strands of collagen occupying less than 10% of the macular or nodular area; 2+, collagen occupying 11–30% of macular or nodular area; 3+, collagen 31–74%; 4+, over 75%.

Goblet Cell Ratio in Peripheral Airways as an Index of Chronic Bronchitis. In individuals without pulmonary disease, bronchioles and small peripheral bronchi have none or only rare goblet cells in their lining epithelium (11). The ratio of goblet to other lining cells increases with chronic bronchitis and bronchiolitis (11). In the present study, goblet and other lining cells were counted in each of 8–20 small peripheral airways in each miner and control case (4, 5, 7). An index of bronchitis was developed by dividing the number of goblet cells in an airway by the total number of epithelial lining cells. A mean index was calculated for each case and for appropriate groups of cases. In no instance was the mean ratio greater than 1/400 in any of the control cases.

Emphysema Index. Emphysema was evaluated by measuring the percent of lung tissue comprised of abnormal air space by the aforementioned microscopic technique of Dunnill (10). This particular measurement was made only on bituminous miners.

Index for Chronic Cor Pulmonale. In each hospital, cardiac right ventricular wall thickness was recorded from each miner's autopsy protocol and for a like number of control males of the same age who had no chronic pulmonary or cardiac valvular disease. An index of chronic cor pulmonale was then calculated for each group of miners by dividing their mean value for right ventricular thickness by the mean value found in the matched controls (8). As individual pathologists differ somewhat in their manner of measuring right ventricular thickness, care was taken to match the number of measurements on miners by an individual pathologist with a like number of measurements by that same pathologist on nonminer control cases.

Quantitative Measurements on Pulmonary Arteries and Arterioles (8).
In all cases, lung tissue was sectioned uniformly at 5μ. Sections were
stained with Verhoeff and Van Gieson's stains. Using a camera lucida
and planimeter under conditions of constant magnification, relative cross
sectional areas of arterial medial circular muscle and intima and any
other elements in the media not comprised of circular muscle were determined in pulmonary muscular arteries under $150\text{-}\mu$ diameter. A percent
of pulmonary artery walls comprised of noncircular muscle was calculated for each case. In the smaller group of 10 miners who had few
arterial intimal abnormalities, relative cross sectional areas of intimal
nuclei and medial nuclei were also determined.

In these latter 10 miners, serial sections over a distance of 2–5 mm were
used to trace individual arteries in and out of coal dust macules. Arteries
measured were divided into two groups depending on whether they were
inside or outside the coal dust macules. The area of individual arterial
intimal nuclei was almost identical in arteries inside and outside the
macules. As vessels were selected which had no proliferative lesions, the
total area of these intimal nuclei was used as an internal standard to
which the area of the artery's media could be compared. The following
ratio was adopted as a measure of the relative area of medial smooth
muscle present in individual arteries: area of arterial media/total area
of intimal nuclei. Since the media of the arteries in question had no visible
collagen or other abnormal tissue, a large ratio indicates a large medial
muscle mass and a small ratio a small muscle mass. In each case, a mean
ratio was determined for pulmonary arteries below 100μ diameter both
inside and outside the coal dust macules.

Results

Right ventricular hypertrophy as evidence of chronic cor pulmonale
appeared in bituminous miners over the age of 50 and was more striking
after age 60 (Table I). It appeared with less than 20 years of mining
experience and became rather severe after 30 or more years of exposure
(Table II). Values for abnormal air space indicate progressively more
emphysema after age 50, but the destructive process can develop with
less than 20 years of underground mining exposure (Tables I and II,
Fig. 1). The volume, crystal and collagen content of dust macules increased with age and duration of underground exposure (Tables I and
II). The collagen content of the dust macules increased with increasing
concentrations of visible silica crystals (Table III). As manifestations of
chronic bronchitis and bronchiolitis, airway goblet cell ratios increased
with age but not necessarily with longer exposure to mine dust (Tables
I and II). Miners with dyspnea had a greater degree of chronic cor

TABLE I

QUANTITATIVE MEASUREMENTS OF LUNG STRUCTURE IN BITUMINOUS MINERS OF VARIOUS AGES[a]

Structural measurement	Ages (years)					Controls (all ages)
	30–49	50–59	60–69	70–79	80+	
Right ventricular thickness (% of control thickness)	102 ± 24	145 ± 54	170 ± 85	159 ± 57	155 ± 68	100 ± 21
Emphysema index						
Lung comprised of abnormal air space (%)	9 ± 5	23 ± 11	28 ± 10	31 ± 10	28 ± 12	5 ± 5
Lung comprised of dust macules (%)	0.3 ± 0.3	1.6 ± 2.4	2.4 ± 3.1	2.9 ± 3.3	3.7 ± 4.8	0
Birefringent crystals in dust macules (per 10,000 μ^2)	1.1 ± 0.2	1.6 ± 0.9	2.0 ± 1.6	1.6 ± 1.1	1.8 ± 1.4	0
Collagen content of dust macules (grades)[b]	0.8 ± 1.1	2.0 ± 1.1	2.1 ± 1.1	2.4 ± 1.0	2.3 ± 1.1	0
Ratio of goblet/nongoblet cells in peripheral airways	$1{:}298 \pm 1{:}211$	$1{:}189 \pm 1{:}158$	$1{:}116 \pm 1{:}127$	$1{:}81 \pm 1{:}93$	$1{:}98 \pm 1{:}112$	$1{:}200+$
Cases in group (%)	6	19	28	29	18	—

[a] Reprinted from Naeye and Dellinger (4).

[b] Collagen grades are as follows: 0, no collagen in macule; 1+, collagen less than 10% of macular area; 2+, collagen 11–30%; and 3+, collagen 31–74%.

TABLE II

QUANTITATIVE MEASUREMENTS OF LUNG STRUCTURE IN BITUMINOUS MINERS WITH VARYING OCCUPATIONAL EXPOSURES TO COAL DUST[a]

Structural measurement (±SD)	Exposure to coal dust (years)				Nonminer controls (all ages)
	2–19	20–29	30–39	40+	
Right ventricular thickness (% of control thickness)	144 ± 7	156 ± 74	171 ± 57	176 ± 83	100 ± 21
Emphysema index					
Lung comprised of abnormal air space (%)	26 ± 13	24 ± 12	30 ± 9	29 ± 12	5 ± 5
Lung comprised of dust macules (%)	2.2 ± 1.8	1.0 ± 0.9	2.6 ± 3.0	3.3 ± 4.5	0
Birefringent crystals in dust macules (per 10,000 μ^2)	0.4 ± 0.6	2.1 ± 1.2	1.6 ± 1.0	1.9 ± 1.4	0
Collagen content of dust macules (grades)	1.6 ± 1.6	2.3 ± 1.1	2.1 ± 1.3	2.3 ± 1.1	0
Ratio of goblet/nongoblet cells in peripheral airways	1:85 ± 1:57	1:87 ± 1:73	1:73 ± 1:71	1:114 ± 1:122	1:200+
Cases in group (%)	7	14	23	56	—

[a] Reprinted from Naeye and Dellinger (4).

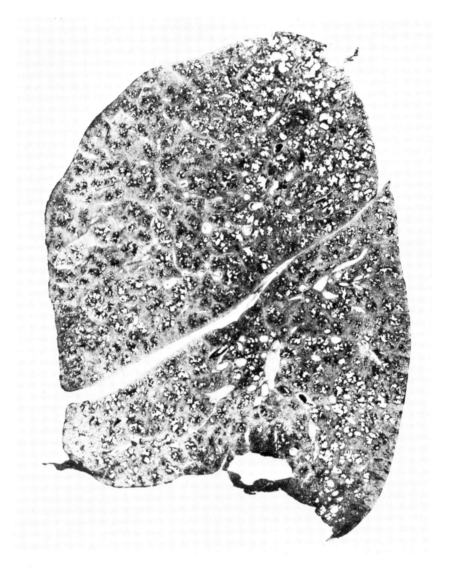

FIG. 1. Coal workers' pneumoconiosis with focal emphysema about the pigmented macules and nodules. Gough section of the lung supplied by Dr. Lorin Kerr.

pulmonale and more emphysema and chronic bronchitis than did those without dyspnea (Table IV). In contrast, the volume, crystal and collagen content of dust macules were similar in the miners with and without dyspnea (Table IV).

Chronic cor pulmonale was most severe in those who had mined the higher-rank bituminous and anthracite coals (Table V). The degree of

TABLE III

RELATIONSHIP BETWEEN CONCENTRATION OF BIREFRINGENT SILICA
CRYSTALS AND COLLAGEN CONTENT OF DUST MACULES IN
BITUMINOUS MINERS[a]

Collagen content of dust (grades)	Birefringent crystals in dust macules (per 10,000 μ^2)	
0–1.5	0.45	$t = 3.26, P < 0.01$
2–4	1.30	

[a] Reprinted from Naeye and Dellinger (4).

cor pulmonale was not related to the amount of noncircular muscle or other abnormal tissue elements in the walls of the small pulmonary arteries (Table V). Most of this noncircular muscle was longitudinally oriented, but there was also an admixture of collagen. The volume, crystal, and collagen content of dust macules increased with coal rank (Table VI). The large, confluent silicotic nodules which were common in the anthracite miners were absent in the bituminous workers, but 44% of this latter group had a few small silicotic nodules (4) (Fig. 2). Sixteen of the anthracite but none of the bituminous miners had grossly visible cavities in at least one pulmonary lobe. Acid-fast bacilli were demonstrated by stain or culture in seven of the men with cavities.

Cor pulmonale was more severe in the miners who smoked. The degree

TABLE IV

QUANTITATIVE MEASUREMENTS OF LUNG STRUCTURE IN BITUMINOUS
MINERS WITH AND WITHOUT CHRONIC DYSPNEA[a]

Structural measurement (ISD)	Bituminous miners		t	$P<$
	With chronic dyspnea	Without dyspnea		
Right ventricular thickness (% of control thickness)	198 ± 74	149 ± 60	2.82	0.01
Emphysema index				
Lung comprised of abnormal air space (%)	32 ± 9	23 ± 10	3.40	0.01
Lung comprised of dust macules (%)	2.81 ± 2.55	4.58 ± 5.31	1.59	0.2
Birefringent crystals in dust macules (per 10,000 μ^2)	2.40 ± 1.46	2.52 ± 1.48	0.29	0.7
Collagen content of dust macules (grades)	2.75 ± 0.76	2.58 ± 0.71	1.00	0.3
Ratio of goblet/nongoblet cells in peripheral airways	1:84 ± 1.89	1:136 ± 1:122	1.38	0.1
Lung disease cases in group (%)	50	50	—	—

[a] Reprinted from Naeye and Dellinger (4).

TABLE V

QUANTITATIVE MEASUREMENTS IN MINERS OF VARIOUS TYPES OF COAL[a]

	Low-rank bituminous	Higher-rank bituminous	High-rank anthracite	Controls
Number of cases	113	58	141	390
Age (years)	68 ± 13	67 ± 10	65 ± 10	66 ± 12
Years of underground exposure	41 ± 12	35 ± 10	33 ± 14	0
Right ventricular thickness (% of controls)	133 ± 51^b	$169 \pm 74^{b,c}$	153 ± 62^b	100 ± 21
Heart weight (grams)	430 ± 116	450 ± 117	431 ± 112	402 ± 91
Percent of pulmonary artery walls comprised of noncircular muscle	55 ± 19	52 ± 14	55 ± 12	50 ± 15

[a] Reprinted from Naeye et al. (5).

[b] P value by comparison with controls less than 0.05.

[c] P value of comparison between adjacent lower rank miners less than 0.05.

of cor pulmonale was not related to the amount of noncircular muscle or other abnormal tissue elements in the walls of their pulmonary muscular arteries (Table VII). For the most part, smoking did not influence the volume, crystal, or collagen content of dust macules (Table VIII). Emphysema was slightly greater in the cigarette smokers, as were anatomic evidences of chronic bronchitis and bronchiolitis (Table VIII).

TABLE VI

QUANTITATIVE MEASUREMENTS OF LUNG STRUCTURE IN MINERS OF VARIOUS TYPES OF COAL[a]

	Low-rank bituminous	Higher-rank bituminous	High-rank anthracite	Controls
Percent of lung comprised of dust macules and nodules	2.0 ± 2.8^b	$3.6 \pm 4.2^{b,c}$	$10.1 \pm 10.8^{b,c}$	0
Birefringent crystals/ 10,000 μ^2 in macules and nodules	0.8 ± 0.9^b	$2.1 \pm 1.6^{b,c}$	$6.7 \pm 6.4^{b,c}$	0
Collagen concentration of macules and nodules (grade)	1.9 ± 1.2^b	$2.6 \pm 0.8^{b,c}$	$3.4 \pm 0.6^{b,c}$	0
Goblet cell nongoblet ratio in peripheral airways	$1:143 \pm 157$	$1:107 \pm 108^{b,c}$	$1:198 \pm 59^b$	$1:200+$

[a] Reprinted from Naeye et al. (5).

[b] P value by comparison with controls less than 0.05.

[c] P value of comparison between adjacent lower rank miners less than 0.05.

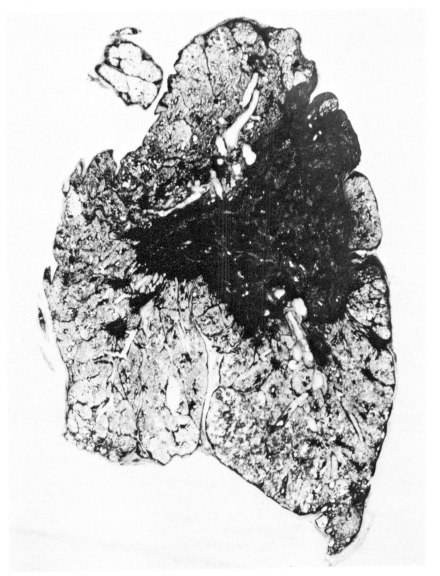

FIG. 2. A pigmented area of massive fibrosis is visible in the upper lung of a 40-year coal worker. This lesion is usually termed progressive massive fibrosis (PMF). Gough section of the lung supplied by Dr. Lorin Kerr.

To further analyze the pathogenesis of chronic cor pulmonale in the miners, the bituminous workers were divided into three subgroups on the basis of cardiac right ventricular wall thickness (Table IX). The degree of cor pulmonale was not related to the amount of noncircular

TABLE VII

THE EFFECTS OF SMOKING ON CARDIAC AND PULMONARY STRUCTURE
OF BITUMINOUS AND ANTHRACITE WORKERS[a]

		Cigarettes			
	Non-smoker	Less than 1 pk/day	1 or more pks	Pipe/cigar	Controls
Right ventricular thickness (% of controls)					
Bituminous	140 ± 60	179 ± 85[b]	186 ± 75[c]	164 ± 57	
Anthracite	157 ± 47	157 ± 52	161 ± 55	154 ± 54	100 ± 21
Heart weight (grams)					
Bituminous	432 ± 64	407 ± 98	439 ± 105	530 ± 209	
Anthracite	413 ± 54	378 ± 97	399 ± 86	378 ± 93	402 ± 91
Years underground					
Bituminous	36 ± 11	38 ± 8	38 ± 10	34 ± 9	
Anthracite	34 ± 7	36 ± 12	32 ± 12	34 ± 16	0
Percent of pulmonary artery walls comprised of noncircular muscle					
Bituminous	51 ± 11	53 ± 16	58 ± 6	47 ± 6	
Anthracite	58 ± 9	57 ± 11	56 ± 10	52 ± 15	50 ± 15
Age (years)					
Bituminous	68 ± 12	66 ± 10	67 ± 9	69 ± 5	
Anthracite	70 ± 9	65 ± 9	60 ± 8[c]	73 ± 8	66 ± 12
Number of cases					
Bituminous	17	19	35	13	
Anthracite	15	13	21	11	390

[a] Reprinted from Naeye et al. (7).
[b] P value by comparison with nonsmokers less than 0.10 (same type coal).
[c] P value by comparison with nonsmokers less than 0.05 (same type coal).

muscle or other abnormal tissue in the walls of the pulmonary arteries (Table IX). Anatomic evidences of arterial thrombosis such as eccentric fibrotic intimal thickening were also virtually absent. The degree of cor pulmonale best correlated with measurements of abnormal air space and goblet cell ratios which reflect emphysema and chronic bronchitis (Table IX). There was no correlation between the volume, crystal, and collagen content of dust macules and the degree of cor pulmonale (Table IX).

To explain the latent pulmonary arterial hypertension observed in some younger miners, one must consider the lesion which antedates emphysema, namely the coal dust macule (Fig. 3). Multiple tissue blocks from the lungs of 10 younger bituminous miners were serially sectioned. Quantitative analysis demonstrated that arterial medial muscle mass significantly increased as these vessels passed through the dust macules. Using the ratio area of arterial media/total area of intimal nuclei, the medial

TABLE VIII

The Effects of Smoking on Pulmonary Structure of Coal Workers[a]

	Nonsmoker	Cigarettes		Pipe/cigar	Controls
		Less than 1 pk/day	1 or more pks		
Percent lung comprised of dust macules					
Bituminous	3.8 ± 2.1	2.9 ± 2.6	4.3 ± 6.6	3.7 ± 2.5	0
Anthracite	9.6 ± 9.4	7.2 ± 7.1	11.7 ± 10.4	16.3 ± 13.5[b]	
Birefringent crystals/10,000 μ^2 in dust macules					
Bituminous	2.0 ± 1.0	1.6 ± 1.6	2.3 ± 1.5	2.2 ± 1.2	0
Anthracite	16.0 ± 8.3	18.4 ± 11.3	14.5 ± 8.6	14.9 ± 8.7	
Collagen content of dust macules					
Bituminous	2.5 ± 0.9	2.4 ± 0.9	2.6 ± 0.6	2.7 ± 0.7	0
Anthracite	3.7 ± 0.5	3.7 ± 0.5	3.8 ± 0.4	3.7 ± 0.5	
Emphysema index: % of lung comprised of abnormal air space					
Bituminous	24.3 ± 7.4	30.1 ± 10.0[b]	30.3 ± 9.6[b]	26.4 ± 9.1	4.8 ± 4.9
Anthracite	—	—	—	—	
Goblet cell/nongoblet cell ratio in airways					
Bituminous	1:151 ± 67	1:96 ± 67[c]	1:97 ± 77[c]	1:90 ± 31[c]	1:200+
Anthracite	1:124 ± 114	1:105 ± 54	1:138 ± 53	1:178 ± 123	

[a] Reprinted from Naeye et al. (7).
[b] P value by comparison with nonsmokers less than 0.05 (same type coal).
[c] P value by comparison with nonsmokers less than 0.10 (same type coal).

TABLE IX

THICKNESS OF CARDIAC RIGHT VENTRICULAR WALL IN PERCENT OF
CONTROLS FROM THE SAME INSTITUTION[a]

Cases were placed in group I when right ventricular thickness was $< 120\%$ of the mean value recorded in the controls; group II, 121–160% of the mean control value; group III, over 160% of the mean control value.

	Group I	Group II	Group III
Right ventricular thickness (% of controls)	96.2 ± 14.5	133.6 ± 14.6^b	223.7 ± 49.5^b
Heart weight (grams)	405.6 ± 93.5	453.2 ± 117.6	466.2 ± 132.9
Age (years)	66.1 ± 11.6	69.1 ± 10.3	69.3 ± 9.8
Underground exposure (years)	37.5 ± 9.8	37.4 ± 13.4	39.3 ± 6.7
Percent of pulmonary artery walls comprised of noncircular muscle	51.7 ± 14.6	53.6 ± 18.8	53.8 ± 15.8
Emphysema index: % of lung comprised of abnormal air space	19.5 ± 9.3	29.6 ± 9.9^b	35.2 ± 8.6^b
Goblet cell nongoblet ratio in peripheral airways	166.7 ± 152.1	78.8 ± 93.2^b	99.3 ± 112.7
Percent of lung comprised of dust macules	2.36 ± 2.71	3.14 ± 3.04	3.03 ± 3.90
Birefringent crystals per 10,000 μ^2 in dust macules	1.37 ± 1.16	1.10 ± 1.14	1.72 ± 1.26
Collagen content of dust macules	2.23 ± 0.70	2.53 ± 0.92	2.20 ± 0.86
Number of cases	76	49	53

[a] Reprinted from Naeye and Laqueur (8).
[b] $P < 0.05$ by comparison with group I.

muscle mass of arteries inside the macules was 2.3 times that of those outside. The increase was mainly due to hypertrophy of arterial medial fibers (8).

Discussion

The pulmonary abnormalities which constitute coal workers' pneumoconiosis can be divided into (a) those related to the dust macule, (b) those associated with the development of bronchitis and emphysema, and (c) those related to massive fibrosis. The primary lesion in CWP is the coal dust macule; it evolves by the incorporation of dust-filled macrophages into the walls of respiratory bronchioles and alveolar ducts. With time, these structures dilate, leading to the development of a halo of focal emphysema about the macule (9). In many miners, silica crystals collect in the macules, the collagen content of the macule being correlated with the crystal concentration (4). This replacement of the macule by collagen appears to be a slow process in most workers. It seems reasonable that

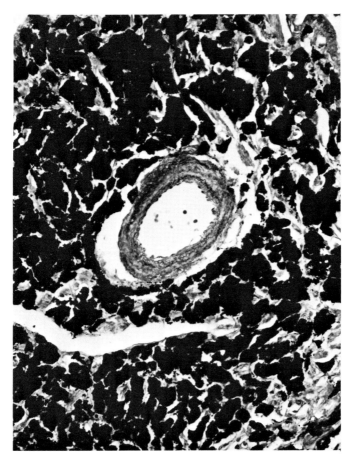

FIG. 3. A muscular pulmonary artery is surrounded by a mantle of pigment in a coal dust macule. Verhoeff's and Van Gieson's stains. ×375.

low concentrations of free silica might induce this change, just as higher concentrations more rapidly induce the whorls of dense collagen typical of the widely recognized silicotic nodule.

Differences in volume, crystal, and collagen content of dust macules explain many of the differences in CWP encountered among miners of differently ranked coals in Pennsylvania and West Virginia (5). The miners of higher-ranked coals have a larger volume of dust macules and silicotic nodules. The macules and nodules in turn have a larger concentration of silica crystals and collagen than do comparable macules and nodules in miners of lower-ranked coal. These findings correlate with a greater prevalence of radiologic abnormalities and a larger request rate for disability benefits from the miners of higher-rank bituminous and anthracite coals (3, 12–15). Since the silica content of all of the coals in question is low, silica exposure in the mines with higher-ranked coals must derive from encounters with rock dust or sand ground under train wheels in the haulage ways (5).

Gough and Nagelschmidt have claimed that carbon itself is an important factor in the pathogenesis of coal workers' pneumoconiosis, but reexamining the data of Nagelschmidt, Pratt has concluded that silica is more important than carbon in the disorder (16–19). In our own studies, the actual volume of coal dust retained in the lungs (largely carbon) seems to have only a small effect on the development of cor pulmonale and the symptoms of pulmonary insufficiency (4, 8). Thus, the association between severity of CWP and rank of coal seems fortuitous, the more important factor being the encounter with free silica (5). Trace elements in mine dust may also be important in the pathogenesis of CWP, but their role is currently not established (20). Acid-fast bacilli appear to contribute to the massive pulmonary fibrosis encountered in some miners, but the bacteria are probably unimportant in the evolution of CWP in the majority of workers.

Chronic bronchitis and the more generalized forms of emphysema make an important contribution to the development of disability in CWP. In our studies, bituminous miners without dyspnea had as large a volume and collagen content of dust macules as did miners with chronic dyspena (4). Dyspnea was best correlated with emphysema. Dyspneic miners had a significantly greater proportion of their lungs comprised of abnormal air space, a hallmark of emphysema. The pathogenesis of this emphysema may well relate to the chronic cough and bronchiolar goblet-cell hyperplasia found in the dyspneic miners (4). Various factors above ground and underground presumably contribute to this bronchitis and emphysema. The incidence and severity of bronchitis and emphysema increase with miners' age but are less influenced by duration of mining exposure. There is a modest effect of cigarette smoking on bronchitis and emphysema in bituminous workers, but some nonsmoking miners also develop these respiratory disorders (7). Above-ground air pollution may contribute to the development of bronchitis and emphysema in some miners. Both miner and nonminer residents often complain of such air pollution in the Pennsylvania and West Virginia valleys where many of the mines are located. In terms of cough, phlegm, wheezing, and breathlessness, the wives of some Appalachian bituminous miners seem to be nearly as affected as their husbands (3).

More than half of the older bituminous and anthracite miners in the current study had moderate or severe cor pulmonale at death. The cor pulmonale is better correlated with the degree of emphysema than with the volume and direct complications of the primary coal dust macule. Pulmonary vascular abnormalities help to explain this cor pulmonale. Arterioles can be found in the lungs of many miners with emphysema and cor pulmonale (8). The reappearance of these vessels which normally disappear in early postnatal life presumably identifies a site of increased vascular resistance. Longitudinal oriented smooth muscle also appears in the walls of the miners' pulmonary arteries, an abnormality attributed to increased longitudinal stretch in emphysema. Anatomic remnants of destroyed pulmonary arteries are rare in most bituminous miners, but it is likely that many small muscular arteries are destroyed as collagen replaces the dust macules in many older workers (8). Remnants of larger occluded arteries are easily seen in the areas of massive fibrosis in many anthracite miners. Pulmonary arterial thrombi have been reported in some European miners but were almost absent in the current study (8, 9, 21).

It is not so easy to explain the mild pulmonary arterial hypertension observed in some younger miners who have little or no emphysema (2). Smooth muscle cells in their small pulmonary arteries hypertrophy as the vessels pass through the mantle of coal dust in the dust macules. If increased vasomotion is the stimulus for this hypertrophy, the macules may well be the site of increased vascular resistance in such miners (8). Increased vascular resistance at this site would also help explain the increased dead space ventilation, decreased diffusing capacity, and dyspnea on exertion observed in some of these younger miners (2).

Summary

A quantitative, morphologic study was undertaken of lung and heart structure on 322 Appalachian miners who were classified by age, duration of mining exposure, rank of coal mined, and smoking habits. Right ventricular hypertrophy as evidence of cor pulmonale was common after age 50. The volume of macular dust lesions, including associated silica crystals, fibrosis, and focal emphysema, increased with age. These dust lesions did not seem solely responsible for dyspnea. Miners with dyspnea also had a generalized form of emphysema. Smoking has a moderate effect on the development of bronchitis and emphysema in bituminous miners but little obvious effect in anthracite workers. The association of pneumoconiosis with coal rank in Appalachia was found to be fortuitous; the prevalence and severity of the disease appears related to varying exposure to silica, chronic bronchitis, and emphysema.

REFERENCES

1. Morgan, W. K. C. (1968). *Amer. Rev. Resp. Dis.* **98**, 306.
2. Rasmussen, D. L., *et al.* (1968). *Amer. Rev. Resp. Dis.* **98**, 658.
3. Lainhart, W. S., *et al.* (1969). *Pub. Health. Ser. Publ.* 2000.
4. Naeye, R. L., and Dellinger, W. S. (1970). *Amer. J. Pathol.* **58**, 557.
5. Naeye, R. L., Mahon, J. K., and Dellinger, W. S. (1971). *Amer. Rev. Resp. Dis.* **103**, 350.
6. "Standard Specifications for Classification of Coals by Rank, Standard D388-66" (1967). Amer. Soc. Testing Material, Philadelphia, Pa. Part 19.
7. Naeye, R. L., Mahon, J. K., and Dellinger, W. S. (1971). *Arch. Environ. Health* **22**, 190.
8. Naeye, R. L., and Laqueur, W. A. (1970). *Arch. Pathol.* **90**, 487.
9. Heppleston, A. G. (1953). *J. Pathol. Bacteriol.* **66**, 235.
10. Dunnill, M. S. (1964). *Thorax* **19**, 443.
11. Reid, L. (1968). "Bronchial Mucus Production in Health and Disease in the Lung" (A. Liebow, ed.). Williams & Wilkins, New York.
12. Lieben, J., Pendergrass, E. G., and McBride, W. W. (1961). *J. Occup. Med.* **3**, 493.
13. McBride, W. W., Pendergrass, E. G., and Lieben, J. (1963). *J. Occup. Med.* **5**, 365.
14. Enterline, P. (1967). *Arch. Environ. Health* **14**, 189.
15. Hyatt, R. E., Kistin, A D., and Mahan, T. K. (1964). *Amer. Rev. Resp. Dis.* **89**, 387.
16. Watson, A. J., *et al.* (1958). *Brit. J. Ind. Med.* **16**, 274.
17. Nagelschmidt, G. (1965). *Amer. Ind. Hyg. Ass. J.* **26**, 1.
18. Pratt, P. C. (1968). *Arch. Environ. Health* **17**, 836.
19. Pratt, P. C. (1968). *Arch. Environ. Health* **16**, 734.
20. Crable, J. V., *et al.* (1968). *Amer. Ind. Hyg. Ass. J.* **29**, 106.
21. Gough, J. (1947). *Occup. Med.* **4**, 86.

7

Roentgenologic Manifestations

*Eugene P. Pendergrass, William S. Lainhart, Leonard J. Bristol,
Benjamin Felson, and George Jacobson*

For the purposes of this presentation it is agreed that pneumoconiosis
should be defined in anatomical terms: Pneumoconiosis is the accumulation of dust in the lungs and the tissue reaction to its presence; the inhalation of coal mine dust is the cause of *coal workers'* pneumoconiosis,
and it can be detected in life by means of an abnormal roentgenographic
pattern and a positive history of dust exposure while working in soft-coal
mines (1).

Pneumoconiosis is a disease in which the radiologist should play the
dominant role in diagnosis and elucidation of the natural history (2). That
opportunity has been enhanced as a result of suggested changes in recording the manifestations of the various patterns of anatomic changes
in the chest (Figs. 17 and 18).

ESSENTIALS OF CHEST RADIOGRAPHY (3)

The most desirable chest radiograph for the study of the pneumoconioses or other pulmonary disease is one in which the lung is shown in
greatest detail. Although it is important to visualize the mediastinal
structures, it is most difficult to obtain a chest radiograph in which both
the lungs and mediastinum are seen equally well. A film in which the
vertebral bodies are faintly visible through the heart shadow will ordi-
narily be adequate for the study of pulmonary detail and also will provide acceptable visualization of the mediastinum.

The maximum information can be obtained from radiographs which have a broad range of contrast, i.e., a long grey scale. High-contrast radiographs should be avoided.

EQUIPMENT

The installation and maintenance of the radiographic equipment is of the greatest importance. The electric power source should be independent of other users. It must be of adequate capacity and should be subject to no more than a 5% fluctuation. The radiographic unit must be carefully calibrated at the time of installation and should be recalibrated periodically. Preventive maintenance at regular intervals, preferably by factory trained personnel, is strongly recommended.

The generator should have a minimum capacity of 300 mA at 125 kV(peak). A generator with a capacity of 150 kV(peak) is strongly recommended. The generator must be full-wave rectified. It should be equipped with an accurate timer (±1%) capable of minimum exposure of no more than 10 mseconds.

A rotating anode tube is essential. It should have as small a focal spot as feasible for the anticipated load, but in no instance should this exceed 2 mm in diameter.

A total filtration, inherent and added, of the primary X-ray beam should be the equivalent of at least 2.5 mm of aluminum.

The radiation should be confined by means of a collimator to the portion of the subject to be examined. This will not only decrease radiation hazard, but will improve detail by reducing scattered radiation. The collimator should have an adjustable diaphragm and a light beam for centering, and it should be designed so the projected field cannot exceed the size of the film. Evidence of collimation should be visible at the edges of the film as "cone cuts."

Medium speed (par speed) intensifying screens should be used. They provide the best compromise between sharp definition and short exposure. The cassettes in use must all contain screens of the same speed and must be checked periodically for screen cleanliness, contact, and defects.

The X-ray film should be of a general purpose type and of medium sensitivity. High-speed film is not recommended. The film should be no larger than needed to cover both lungs, including the costophrenic angles.

When using kilovoltages of 80 and above, reduction of secondary radiation by a grid or other means is essential. A 10:1, 100 line/in. fixed grid or an air-gap of 8 in. with an 8-ft focal-spot–film distance may be used.

Automatic processing should be employed whenever possible. If only manual processing is available, a constant time–temperature technique must be followed meticulously. An improper exposure cannot be corrected by improper processing.

Further improvement in radiographic quality may be expected with the use of a three-phase generator or other means of increasing the effective photon energy, high-speed rotating anode tubes, smaller focal spots, finer grain film, etc.

TECHNIQUE

Correct centering of the X-ray tube and careful positioning of the subject are of great importance for the proper visualization of anatomic structures and comparison of serial examinations. For the P-A projection, the X-ray tube should be centered to the center of the film and the beam directed horizontally. The shoulders should be positioned so the scapulae are outside the lungs. The exposure should be made at full inspiration and made immediately after this has been reached to avoid the Valsalva effect. It is desirable, but not essential, that all the clothes above the waist be removed.

The focal-spot–film distance should be fixed between 5 and 6 ft (approximately 1.5 and 2.0 m).

For the reasons given above, a variable high kilovoltage, constant mA-second technique is recommended. Exposure factors employed may vary somewhat with each generator and tube. The highest range of kilovoltage and shortest range of mA-second obtainable should be used. For the average subject, with an A-P chest diameter between 21 and 23 cm, the usual exposure factors will be 5 mA-second at approxi-

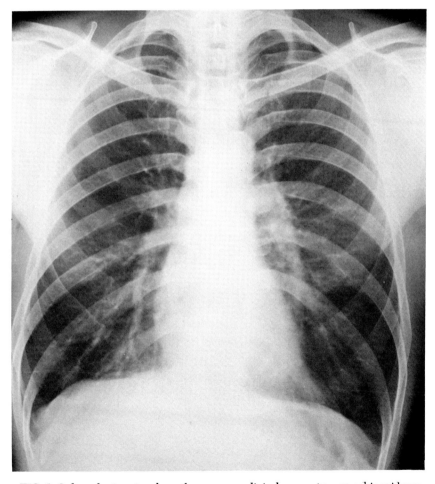

FIG. 1. Soft-coal miner in whom there was no clinical or roentgenographic evidence of pneumoconiosis. Note the pattern of the major vascular components, arteries and veins. Many of the small vessels do not produce a pattern that can be seen. This chest study is characterized as Category 0.

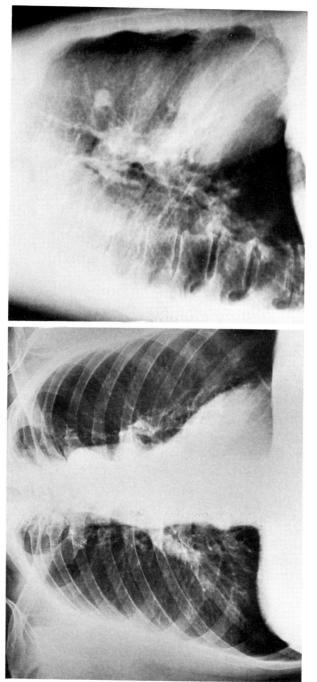

FIG. 2. Adenosquamous carcinoma of the left upper lobe in a 65-year-old white man. There were no symptoms, and the lesion was found in a routine chest examination which fortunately included posteroanterior and left lateral views. In the P-A roentgenogram, the lesion was not seen because its shadow was superimposed on the shadow of the left hilum. The shadow of the lesion is readily seen in the lateral view.

mately 125 kV(peak). The recommended exposure time is 1/60 (0.017) second.* It should not exceed 1/30 (0.032) second. With chests of larger diameter, additional exposure is obtained by increasing the kilovoltage. The mA-second is increased only when the kilovoltage required to give a proper exposure exceeds the capability of the generator or X-ray tube. With focal-spot–film distances of less than 6 ft (2.0 m) the technique should be adjusted by decreasing the mA-second.

With the low-kilovoltage technique, the exposure factors for the average subject are approximately 300 mA × 0.05 second (15 mA-second) at 75 kV. For larger subjects, either the mA-second or the kilovoltage are increased.

Phototimers are inaccurate with exposures of less than 0.03 second and are not recommended with the technique suggested above. However, phototiming can be very useful with exposure of longer duration.

What Roentgenograms Should be Made?

Survey radiographic examinations oftentimes are limited to a single posteroanterior (P-A) roentgenogram made in the erect posture (Fig. 1). On occasion, other exposures may be used; P-A view in expiration and inspiration; anteroposterior (A-P) view in inspiration; and right and left lateral views. Each view provides additional and sometimes very important information. One real value of stereoscopic P-A views is that one has two views made within a few seconds of each other. If one places the films side by side one may note the variation in the vascular pattern and one may find small opacities that resemble a pattern of pneumoconiosis on one roentgenogram and not in the other. In many instances, especially when emphysema is present, P-A views made in inspiration and expiration are helpful in demonstrating small opacities which are less prominent in the inspiratory roentgenogram. With pleural calcification and thickening, the lateral view provides important information in addition to that found in the P-A roentgenogram. Small parenchymal lesions 1–3 cm in size may not be recognized in P-A roentgenograms when their shadows are superimposed upon those of the hila, but they are readily detected in the lateral view (Fig. 2).

ROENTGENOGRAPHIC PATTERNS OF COAL WORKERS' PNEUMOCONIOSIS

The roentgenographic changes in coal workers' pneumoconiosis seen in the United States involves the lungs, the pleura, and their supporting structures. My own experience has largely been with coal miners in Alabama, Appalachia, Illinois, Indiana, Pennsylvania, and Utah (4–6).

---

* Based on 60-cps current. For 50-cps current, exposure times are 1/50 (0.02) and 1/25 (0.04) second.

Cardiac abnormalities may occur, but the roentgen examination without elaborate contrast studies does not contribute very much.

The patterns of small and large opacities in coal workers' pneumoconiosis in many instances are similar to those seen in anthracosilicosis. In others, the shadow pattern of abnormal changes, largely, are seen in the lower two-thirds of the lung fields (5).

Emphysema, as a rule, is not well portrayed in P-A roentgenograms of coal workers' pneumoconiosis.

Pleural thickening is often seen. It occurs along the periphery and in the interlobar fissures. In most instances it is a generalized thickening and not plaque-like. Calcification of the pleura occurs, and it may be very slight or extensive. As far as we have been able to discover, there has not been an exposure to asbestos dust in those instances where calcified pleura was found in coal workers' pneumoconiosis (7, 8).

Aims and Principles of the UICC (U/C) Classification (Table I)

This classification is a modification of the ILO 1958 scheme and others (9). Quoting freely from the original manuscript (10), this classification:

as far as possible is purely descriptive of radiographic appearances and does not use interpretive words such as "fibrosis" or "infection" which already have definitions in terms of pathology;

describes the natural history of the changes produced by all dusts as far as is known, but it avoids the use of terms such as "early stages," "progressive," or "final";

provides a system of recording qualitatively and semiqualitatively (with the help of verbal descriptions and standard films) different features of the film which can be separately assessed and graded. It provides a code that permits a brief description of the important radiographic features of the pneumoconioses.

General Description of the Classification

The ILO 1958 scheme divided the opacities in the lung fields (lung parenchyma) into "small" and "large." The U/C scheme retains that main subdivision but further divides the small opacities into "rounded" and "irregular," and the large opacities into "well defined" and "ill defined." The ILO scheme recorded pleural changes with a symbol "pl." The U/C scheme brings the pleural changes into the main classification, with a subdivision "calcified" and "noncalcified."* It also records the presence of a poorly defined cardiac outline and diaphragm within the main scheme but retains the symbol "co" (abnormal cardiac shape) as defined in the ILO scheme and its later modification by the U. S. Public Health Service (9) (See Chapter 3, Fig. 1).

Provision has been made for the separate recording of three features for each variable (Figs. 14 and 15):

1. *Type:* for example, small or large, rounded or irregular, calcified, etc.;

2. *Profusion:* the number of opacities (rounded or irregular) per unit area, e.g., per zone (see below). The word *profusion* is used in preference to density because this latter word is also used radiologically to describe the radiopacity of a shadow. The profusion is graded on a basic four-point scale—0, 1, 2, 3—with a means of increasing this to a twelve-point scale when greater precision is required.

3. *Extent:* the area (number of zones) of the lung field affected or length, as in the case of cardiac border involvement. This also provides information about the site of abnormality, which may later be of value.

In the ILO 1958 scheme, category 1 of small opacities was defined in terms of the number of rib spaces involved—a measure of extent. Categories 2 and 3 included factors of both extent and of profusion. One of the criticisms of the ILO 1958 scheme was that it failed to provide for the classification of a film with definite but very sparse rounded opacities seen in more than two rib spaces. That criticism is met in the U/C scheme.

The classification recognizes the existence of a continuum of change from complete normality to the most advanced category or grade in the recorded features. For example, with regard to small opacities a film may be correctly classified as category 0 if there are no opacities seen or if it is thought to show a few which are not sufficiently definite or numerous to reach the definition of category 1 (Table I). No sudden step from normality to abnormality is implied at the 0–1 boundary.

Details of the Classification (10)

SMALL OPACITIES

These are classified as in the ILO 1958 scheme modified by the U. S. Public Health Service, with some further alteration of the verbal definitions.

---

* The use of the word "calcified" is at variance with the general principle of not using interpretive words, but it was accepted because of its wide utilization in radiology.

TABLE I

UICC/Cincinnati Classification of Radiographic Appearances of Pneumoconioses[a]

		Codes	Definitions
Small opacities	Rounded profusion		The category of profusion is based on assessment of the concentration of opacities in the affected zones. The standard films define the mid-categories.
		0/– 0/0 0/1	Category 0—small rounded opacities absent or less profuse than in category 1
		1/0 1/1 1/2	Category 1—small rounded opacities definitely present but relatively few in number
		2/1 2/2 2/3	Category 2—small rounded opacities numerous. The normal lung markings are usually still visible.
		3/2 3/3 3/4	Category 3—small rounded opacities very numerous. The normal lung markings are partly or totally obscured.
	Type	p q r	The nodules are classified according to the approximate diameter of the predominant opacities.
			p—rounded opacities up to about 1.5 mm diameter
			q—rounded opacities exceeding about 1.5 mm and up to about 3 mm diameter
			r—rounded opacities exceeding about 3 mm and up to about 10 mm diameter
	Extent	Lung zones	The zones in which the opacities are seen are recorded. Each lung is divided into thirds—upper, middle, lower zones. Thus a maximum of six zones can be affected.
	Irregular profusion		The category of profusion is based on assessment of the concentration of opacities in the affected zones. The standard films define the mid-categories.
		0/– 0/0 0/1	Category 0—small irregular opacities absent or less profuse than in category 1

	1/0 1/1 1/2	Category 1—small irregular opacities definitely present but relatively few in number The normal lung markings are usually visible.
	2/1 2/2 2/3	Category 2—small irregular opacities numerous The normal lung markings are usually partly obscured.
	3/2 3/3 3/4	Category 3—small irregular opacities very numerous The normal lung markings are usually totally obscured.
Type	s t u	Since the opacities are irregular, the dimensions used for rounded opacities cannot be used, but they can be roughly divided into three types. s—fine irregular or linear opacities t—medium irregular opacities u—coarse (blotchy) irregular opacities
Extent	Lung zones	The zones in which the opacities are seen are recorded. Each lung is divided into thirds—upper, middle, lower zones—as for rounded opacities.
Large opacities — Size	A B C	Category A—an opacity with greatest diameter between 1 cm and 5 cm, or several such opacities the sum of whose greatest diameters does not exceed 5 cm Category B—one or more opacities larger or more numerous than those in category A, whose combined area does not exceed one-third of the area of the right lung Category C—one or more large opacities whose combined area exceeds one-third of the area of the right lung
Type	wd id	As well as the letter "A," "B," or "C," the abbreviation "wd" or "id" should be used to indicate whether the opacities are well defined or ill defined.

(Continued)

TABLE I (*Continued*)

		Codes		Definitions
Other features	Pleural thickening	Right	Left	
	Costophrenic angle			Obliteration of the costophrenic angle is recorded separately from thickening over other sites. A lower limit standard film is provided.
	Other sites	1 2	3	Grade 0—not present or less than grade 1
				Grade 1—up to 5 mm thick and not exceeding one-half of the projection of one lateral chest wall. A lower limit standard film is provided.
				Grade 2—more than 5 mm thick and up to one-half of the projection of one lateral chest wall or up to 5 mm thick and exceeding one-half of the projection of one lateral chest wall
				Grade 3—more than 5 mm thick and exceeding more than one-half of the projection of one lateral chest wall
	Diaphragm	Right	Left	
	Ill defined			The lower limit is one-third of the affected hemidiaphragm. A lower limit standard film is provided.
	Cardiac outline			
	Ill defined (shagginess)	1 2	3	Grade 0—up to one-third of the length of the left cardiac border or equivalent
				Grade 1—above one-third and up to two-thirds of the length of the left cardiac border or equivalent
				Grade 2—above two-thirds and up to the whole length of the left cardiac border or equivalent

Grade 3—more than the whole length of the left cardiac border or equivalent

Pleural calcification

Diaphragm   1   2   3
Walls
Other sites

Grade 0—no pleural calcification seen
Grade 1—one or more areas of pleural calcification, the sum of whose greatest diameters does not exceed 2 cm
Grade 2—one or more areas of pleural calcification, the sum of whose greatest diameters exceeds 2 cm but does not exceed 10 cm
Grade 3—one or more areas of pleural calcification, the sum of whose greatest diameters exceeds 10 cm

Other symbols:
Obligatory
ca—suspect cancer of lung or pleura
co—abnormality of cardiac size or shape
cp—suspect cor pulmonale
es—eggshell calcification of hilar or mediastinal lymph nodes
tba—opacities suggestive of active clinically significant tuberculosis
od—other significant disease. This includes disease not related to dust exposure, e.g., surgical or traumatic damage to chest walls, bronchiectasis, etc.

Optional
ax—coalescence of small rounded pneumoconiotic opacities
bu—bullae
cn—calcification in small parenchymal opacities
cv—cavity
di—marked distortion of the intrathoracic organs
em—marked emphysema
hi—marked enlargement of hilar shadows
ho—honeycomb lung
k—Kerley (septal) lines
px—pneumothorax
rl—pneumoconiosis modified by rheumatoid process
tb—inactive tuberculosis

a U/C Classification of Radiographic Appearances of Pneumoconiosis was arranged into a table by the American College of Radiology for its teaching seminar in Washington, D. C., 13–14 June 1970.

Type: The nodules are classified according to the approximate diameter of the predominant opacities. Strict adherence to measurement is not intended.

p = rounded opacities up to about 1.5 mm in diameter (Figs. 3 and 4)
q = rounded opacities exceeding about 1.5 mm and up to about 3 mm in diameter (Fig. 5)
r = rounded opacities exceeding about 3 mm in diameter up to about 10 mm in diameter (Fig. 6)

Profusion: The standard films define the midcategories.

Category 0—small rounded opacities absent or less profuse than in category 1
Category 1—small rounded opacities definitely present but relatively few in number. The normal lung markings (vascular pattern) are usually visible.

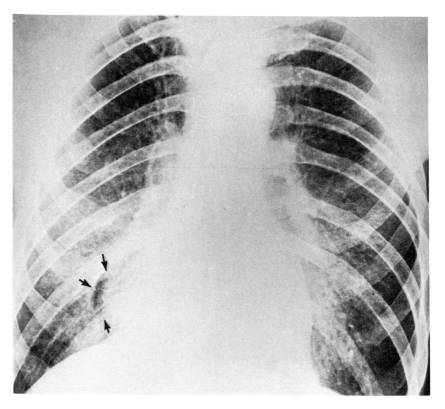

FIG. 3. Coal workers' pneumoconiosis, category 3 p and u in a West Virginia coal miner. The profusion of small opacities is 3/4, and it is difficult to identify the individual rounded and irregular small opacities. See Fig. 4. The cardiac outlines, right and left, are ill defined, probably grade 3. There is a medium sized bulla in right lower lobe indicated by arrows.

Category 2—small rounded opacities numerous. The normal lung markings are usually still visible.

Category 3—small rounded opacities very numerous. The normal lung markings are partly or totally obscured.

The category of profusion is based not on extent, but only on the concentration of opacities in the affected zones.

Extent (10): The specific zones in which the opacities are seen are recorded. Each lung field is divided into thirds—upper, middle, and lower zones. Thus, there can be a maximum of six zones affected.

Notes (10)

(1) *q* and *r* are used in place of *m* and *n* of the ILO 1958 scheme because of

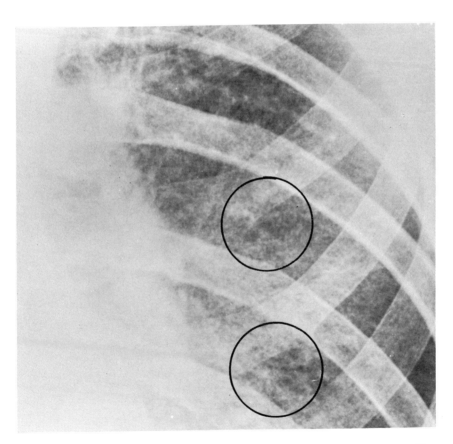

FIG. 4. Same case as Fig. 3. Close-up of the left middle lung. The *p* opacities (upper circle) predominate, and it is difficult to identify the irregular opacities (lower circle) *u* on the lower interspaces. The left cardiac border is ill defined.

phonetic and scriptory errors caused by using *m* and *n*. No change of definition is entailed.

(2) In category 1, small rounded opacities are commonly seen in the upper and middle zones but may occur in any zones or in one lung only. Rarely in categories 2 and 3 are they present in only one lung.

(3) There is evidence (11–14) that subdivision into finer grades than the four categories—0, 1, 2, 3—is possible without the use of extra standard films and that it conveys extra information for epidemiological purposes. The instructions are to

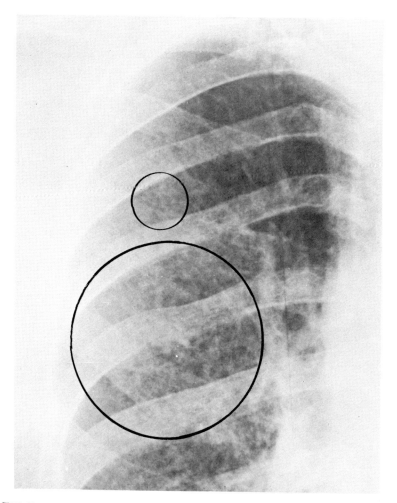

FIG. 5. Small rounded and irregular opacities in coal workers' pneumoconiosis. The rounded opacities in the fourth interspace posteriorly (small circle) are largely *p* and *q*. The irregular opacities in the fifth and sixth interspaces (large circle) are largely the *t* type ("circular," "network," "linear").

classify the film in the usual way into one of the four categories and, if during the process a neighboring category is considered as a serious alternative, to record this after the formal category. Thus category 2/1 is a film which is category 2 but category 1 was seriously considered as an alternative. The film which is without doubt a category 2, i.e., a midcategory closely similar in profusion to the standard film, would be classified as 2/2. In films within category 0 a subdivision is also possible. Thus, category 0/1 is a film which is category 0 but category 1 was seriously considered. Category 0/0 is a normal film without small opacities. Occasionally films look exceptionally "normal," i.e., exceptional clarity of the normal architecture. These "barn door" normal films are usually, though not exclusively, from young individuals. Provision for these is made by the category 0/—. Thus the formal four-point scale becomes a twelve-point scale: 0/—, 0/0, 0/1, 1/0, 1/1, 1/2, 2/1, 2/2, 2/3, 3/2, 3/3, 3/4. In practice this elaborated scale takes no longer than the four-point system, and it is easier for the reader, as his doubts about the borderline films are quickly recorded (Figs. 17 and 18).

SMALL IRREGULAR OPACITIES (10)

This category is the main new feature of the classification. The term is used to describe features which in other schemes have been called

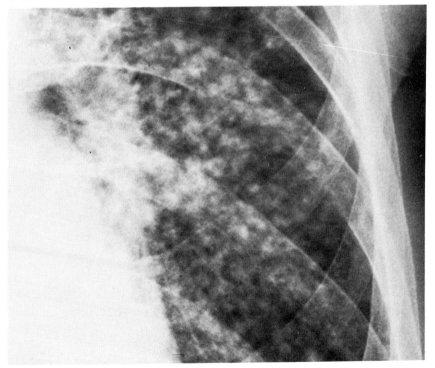

FIG. 6. Coal workers' pneumoconiosis with a pattern of small rounded opacities, *r*. As usual there are small irregular opacities in the same field; the *r* opacities are more dominant.

linear, reticular, fibrotic, network, and honeycomb (Fig. 7). It includes films which would be classified as L in the ILO 1958 scheme and also some, but not all, films formerly read as Z. Small irregular opacities are of varying thickness, shape, and density and often have a curved or linear appearance. They tend to obscure the normal lung architecture (vascular pattern), particularly when present in considerable profusion. Hence, obscuration of normal lung architecture is a feature of the higher categories of both small "rounded" and small "irregular" opacities.

Type: On account of the irregularity of the opacities, the dimensions used for the rounded opacities cannot be applied, but to conform to the general scheme, the types may be roughly divided into three:

s = fine irregular or linear opacities
t = medium thick irregular opacities (Fig. 8)
u = coarse (blotchy) irregular opacities (Fig. 9)

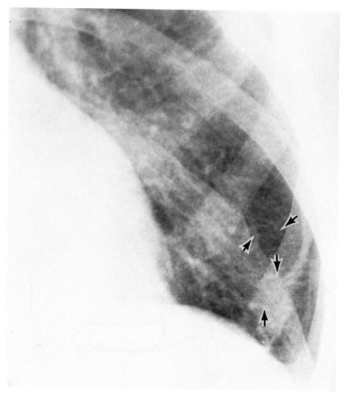

FIG. 7. Coal workers' pneumoconiosis in a Pennsylvania soft-coal miner with small rounded opacities, p; and straight B lines (Kerley) and curvilinear patterns, u. The rounded opacities p (upper two arrows) are not well seen in the illustration. The lines and irregular opacities are well illustrated in the area of the lower arrows.

Assessment is made of the predominant type of small irregular opacity by comparison with the appropriate standard film.

Profusion: The standard films define the midcategories.

Category 0—small irregular opacities absent or less profuse than in category 1
Category 1—small irregular opacities definitely present but relatively sparse. The normal lung markings are usually visible.
Category 2—small irregular opacities numerous. The normal lung markings are usually partly obscured.
Category 3—small irregular opacities very numerous. The normal lung markings are usually totally obscured.

The category of profusion is based not on extent, but only on the concentration of opacities in the affected zones.

Extent (10): The specific zones in which the irregular opacities are seen are recorded. Each lung is divided into thirds—upper, middle, and lower zones, as for rounded opacities.

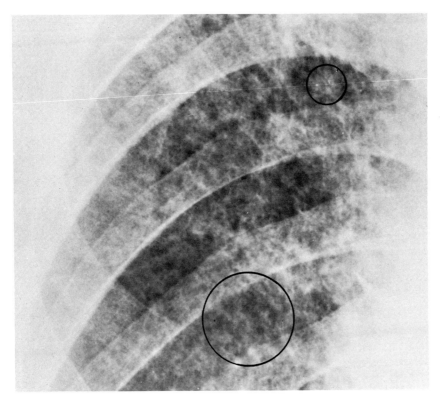

FIG. 8. Right upper lobe of a West Virginia miner with coal workers' pneumoconiosis to illustrate small irregular opacities *u* (lower circle) and ax (upper small circle).

Murphy, in a special study of asbestosis, used two zones, upper and lower, in each lung field (15).

Notes (*10*)

(1) The types *s*, *t*, and *u* are less well differentiated than the *p*, *q*, *r* sequence of small rounded opacities. It is not known whether the subdividing of irregular opacities in this way will be useful, nor was it known when *p*, *m*, and *n* were first suggested that pathological and functional differences existed between the different types. Subsequent research has shown they are meaningful.

(2) In category 1, small irregular opacities are commonly seen in the lower zones, but may occur in any zones or in one lung only.

(3) The differentiation between "rounded" and "irregular" opacities is readily seen by comparing the standard films of each type, but films occur in which both types are seen. It is recommended that both "rounded" and "irregular" should be recorded if both types are clearly seen in the same film. However, further research is needed to show how well they can be differentiated (Figs. 3–9).

(4) Experience in classifying films of mineral dust pneumoconiosis has revealed a

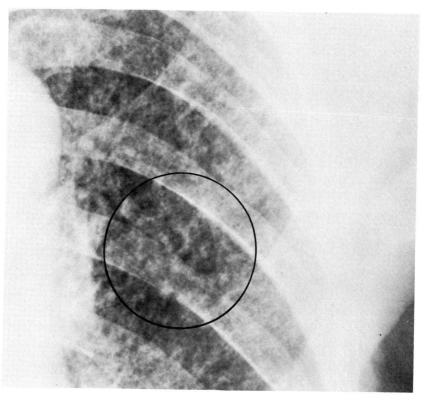

FIG. 9. Same case as Fig. 8. Left upper lobe. Note that *u* opacities (within circle) are more dominant on the left side and *t* opacities on the right. The *q* opacities are seen where the profusion of irregular opacities are less dominant.

small proportion which, though undoubtedly abnormal and probably the result of dust exposure, do not fit well into the ILO classification. The U/C classification provided a means of classifying these as they often fit well into the "small irregular opacities" group.

(5) Where there is a marked difference in profusion in different parts of the lungs, the zones predominantly affected are the ones over which averaging is made.

Large Opacities

The scheme used is that in the ILO 1958 classification, with the additional qualification of "well defined" (wd) and "ill defined" (id). The well-defined large opacities are those covered by A, B, and C in the ILO 1958 system. The ill-defined are those opacities in which the edge is very poorly differentiated from the surrounding lung. Large opacities of that type sometimes occur in advanced asbestosis, but they are also seen in other types of pneumoconiosis. Thus U/C provides a more complete system of recording the features of large opacities.

Category A—an opacity having a diameter exceeding 1 cm and up to and including 5 cm, or several opacities each greater than 1 cm, the sum of whose greatest diameters does not exceed 5 cm (Figs. 10–12)

Category B—one or more opacities larger or more numerous than those in category A whose combined area does not exceed one-third of the right lung field (Fig. 22)

Category C—one or more opacities whose combined area exceed one-third of the right lung field (Fig. 13)

Notes
(1) The abbreviation wd or id should be used to indicate whether the shadows are well or ill defined (Figs. 10 and 13). Reference to the standard films will help to make the differentiation. Sometimes both types should be recorded.
(2) When recording large opacities the type and category of small opacities in the background should also be noted. If small opacities are not seen, a comment to this effect must be recorded (Figs. 17 and 18).

Pleural Thickening (10)

Pleural thickening is classified according to type (diffuse or plaques), site, and extent, but changes which might represent pleural thickening over the diaphragm and cardiac outline are recorded separately, because there is insufficient evidence, especially in cases of asbestosis, to be certain whether the ill-defined outline of the cardiac border (shaggy heart) or diaphragm is the result of pleural thickening or alteration of adjacent lung parenchyma (Fig. 13).

Costophrenic Angle: Obliteration of the costophrenic angle is recorded separately from thickening over other areas because it is so commonly seen in individuals with no history of dust exposure (Fig. 13). A lower-limit standard film is provided. No upper-limit film is used. If the thickening extends further up the chest wall, then the film should be classified as costophrenic angle obliteration *and* pleural thickening, if this is as up to grade 1 or more. Costophrenic angle obliteration is recorded as absent or present, right or left.

Note: Leafing (scalloping) of the diaphragm should not be recorded as costophrenic angle obliteration.

Chest Wall: Pleural thickening is recorded in four grades as follows:

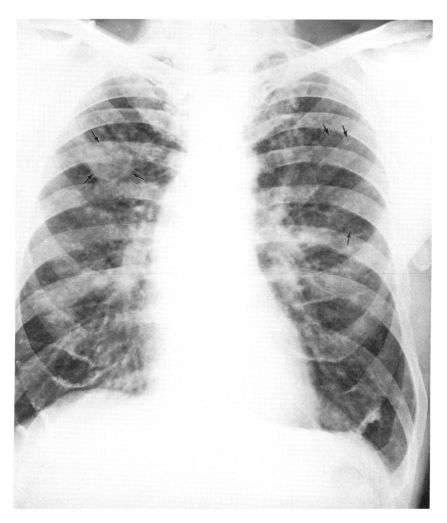

FIG. 10. Coal workers' pneumoconiosis in a Pennsylvania soft-coal miner; category 3 *r* A. The background of small opacities *r* extend throughout both lungs. The large opacity in the right upper lobe "A" is interpreted as evidence of a complicated pneumoconiosis. It is well defined.

Grade 0—not present or less than grade 1
Grade 1—definite pleural thickening up to 5 mm thick which alone or combined
with similar shadows does not exceed half of one chest wall. The standard film is at the lower limit of grade 1.

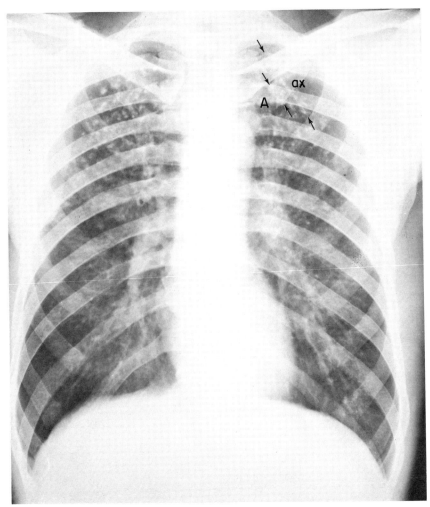

FIG. 11. Coal workers' pneumoconiosis in a Pennsylvania coal miner. Category 2
q A, ax, hi, cn. Many of the small rounded opacities are calcified "cn," but some are
not. There are two conglomerate lesions in the left upper lobe. The oval lesion ap-
proaches the size of Category "A." It seems to be a well-defined large opacity. The
long coalescent lesion is categorized as "ax." When a large opacity is present, it is
not necessary to identify and record ax. It is not known whether the calcification is
due to histoplasmosis or to some other process such as tuberculosis. The hila are
prominent.

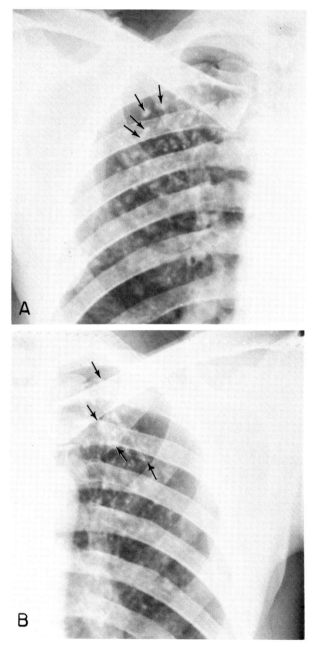

FIG. 12. Same case as Fig. 11. (A) Close-up of the right upper lobe to show the detail of the calcium deposits in the small opacities *q*. (B) Close-up of left upper lobe showing the details of the oval conglomerate opacity, "A" and the long shadow pattern, "ax."

Grade 2—pleural thickening more than 5 mm thick and up to half of one chest wall, *or* less than 5 mm thick if it extends more than the equivalent of one-half of one chest wall. The standard film is at the lower limit of grade 2.

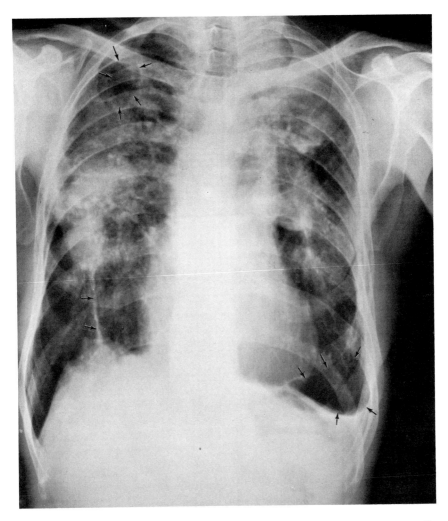

FIG. 13. Coal workers' pneumoconiosis in a Pennsylvania soft-coal miner, 3 *q* C, hi, di, em, pl, and bullae. The small opacities are obscured by the large ill-defined opacities and emphysema. The hila are displaced upward and the heart and aorta to the right. The domes of the diaphragm are distorted. There is a band-like shadow which extends from the large opacity in the right midlung to the dome of the diaphragm (arrows). There is a large bulla in the right apex and in the left costophrenic sulcus (arrows). The left costophrenic sulcus is obliterated, and there is a slight scoliosis. The right cardiac border is partially ill defined.

Grade 3—pleural thickening more than 5 mm thick and extending more than the equivalent of one-half of one chest wall

Note

(1) Do not record the "companion" rib shadows that simulate pleural thickening.

(2) The sharpness of the outline of the pleural thickening varies greatly. In asbestos-exposed workers it may appear as a well-defined band along the lateral chest wall (see Grade 1 standard film) or as a much more wide-spread shadow. The widespread and well-defined forms are recorded together as "diffuse." Occasionally, localized areas of uncalcified pleural thickening—pleural plaques—are seen on the diaphragm or chest wall, and should be recorded as such. The diffuse and localized forms should be considered together when grading pleural thickening.

(3) Pleural thickening on the ventral or posterior walls of the chest may lead to obscuration of the lung fields and may be recognizable on lateral views.

ILL-DEFINED DIAPHRAGM (10)

This is recorded as absent or present and right or left. The lower limit is one-third of the affected hemidiaphragm. A lower-limit standard film is provided.

Note: A single adhesion, scalloping, hernia, eventration, calcification, plaque, and tumor are not included within the term "ill-defined diaphragm."

ILL-DEFINED CARDIAC OUTLINE (10)

Only the length of the cardiac border affected is used for grading. The degree of poorness of definition is not separately recorded. Four grades are used. Regardless of which side is affected, the grading is based on the length of the left heart border.

Grade 0—up to one-third of the left cardiac border or equivalent (Fig. 13)
Grade 1—between one-third and two-thirds of the left cardiac border or equivalent
Grade 2—between two-thirds and the entire left cardiac border or equivalent
Grade 3—more than the left cardiac border (Figs. 3 and 4)

Note

(1) The sharpness of the cardiac border is affected by heart movement and hence the exposure time of the radiograph. If this is the only cause for the irregular cardiac border, do not record it.

(2) Cardiac fat pads are not included in the grading. Grade 1 is set fairly high, so only the more definitely abnormal films will be graded 1 or above.

(3) In asbestos-exposed workers the earliest change in the radiograph may be an ill-defined cardiac outline.

PLEURAL CALCIFICATION (10)

This feature is recorded separately from pleural thickening, the site noted, and whether the calcification is uni- or bilateral. It is also graded with the help of standard films.

Grade 0—no pleural calcification

Grade 1—an area of calcified pleura with greatest diameter not exceeding 2 cm, or a number of such areas, the sum of whose greatest diameters does not exceed 2 cm in length

Grade 2—an area of calcified pleura with greatest diameter exceeding 2 cm and not exceeding 10 cm, or a number of such areas, the sum of whose greatest diameters exceeds 2 cm but not more than 10 cm (Fig. 14)

Grade 3—an area of calcified pleura with greatest diameter exceeding 10 cm or a number of such areas whose sum of greatest diameters exceeds 10 cm [Figs. 15(A) and 15(B)].

Note: Uni- or bilaterality is recorded because calcification due to mineral dusts, including asbestos, is often bilateral, whereas that due to other causes, such as infection and trauma, is more usually unilateral.

ADDITIONAL SYMBOLS (10)

Additional symbols are used as in the ILO 1958 scheme to record features which are not in the main classification. If all symbols are op-

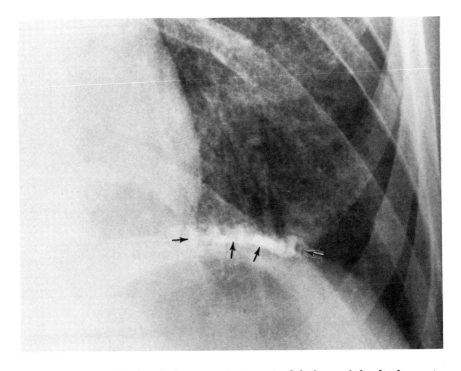

FIG. 14. Calcified pleural plaque, grade 2, on the left dome of the diaphragm in a West Virginia miner who has extensive complicated coal workers' pneumoconiosis. There are numerous small rounded and irregular opacities. The calcified pleural plaque is seen clearly, because the plaque is on the crest of the dome and is recorded in an axial view.

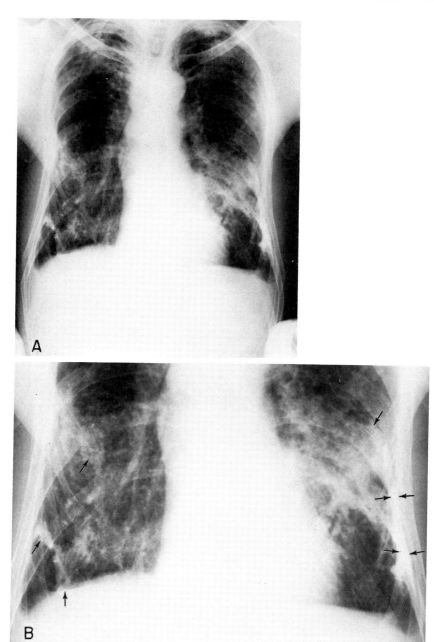

FIG. 15. (A) Extensive calcified pleura, grade 3, along thoracic walls and right dome of the diaphragm in a Pennsylvania soft-coal miner. The small opacities are largely obscured by the calcium deposits. Lateral views oftentimes provide informa-

tional, the recording is usually incomplete. Two groups—obligatory (Fig. 16) and optional—are therefore recommended. See Table I.

GENERAL INSTRUCTIONS (10)

When deciding whether a film is to be classified within the scheme, the following recommendations are made:

(1) Decide if *any* of the changes seen in the pleura or the parenchyma sufficiently resemble the pattern of any of the pneumoconioses to be recorded. If so, proceed with the classification.

(2) If it is probable that *all* the changes seen are the result of some

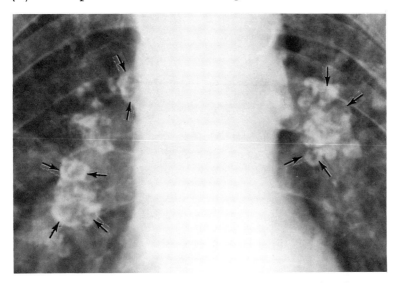

FIG. 16. Coal workers' pneumoconiosis in a Pennsylvania soft-coal miner. Category 3 *r*, hi, es. This illustration is a good example of eggshell calcification in the hila lymph nodes. Eggshell calcification is defined as shell-like calcifications measuring up to 2 mm in thickness present in the peripheral zone of at least two lymph nodes, which may be broken or unbroken, but the ring-like shadow must be complete in at least one node; there may be flecks of calcium in the central portions, and one of the nodes must be at least 1 cm in its greatest diameter.

---

tion not seen in the axial view. This is true particularly where the calcium deposits are on the anterior or posterior chest wall or on the sloping portions of the domes of the diaphragm and are not in a position for axial projections of X-ray radiation in the usual P-A view. (B) Close-up view, which provides more detail. The arrows illustrate the thickness of the pleural calcification along the left lateral chest wall. The large shadows in the lower half of the left and right lung fields are due to calcified pleura on the anterior chest wall (arrows). There is a calcified pleural plaque on the right dome of the diaphragm (arrow).

etiology other than pneumoconiosis, do not classify but record opinion using appropriate symbols and comments.

(3) If changes might be due to pneumoconiosis, classify features, but make a note that other etiology is possible.

In the U/C scheme, unlike the ILO schemes, no provision is made for doubtful pneumoconiosis. This omission is intentional since the scheme is intended principally for epidemiological studies where a "suspect" group contributes little to the information. The provision of a twelve-point scale for both small rounded and small irregular opacities provides a method of classifying radiographs less than category 1.

In epidemiological studies failure to record all readings can be an important source of loss of information. To reduce this to a minimum the recording sheet (Fig. 17) is so designed that at least one entry must be made between each pair of heavy lines. In Fig. 18, ten sketches of the roentgen appearance of lesions in pneumoconiosis are given, together with their corresponding readings.

RADIOLOGIC CONSIDERATIONS (2)

The radiologic problems in the pneumoconioses concerned with the interpretation and evaluation of the shadow patterns of intrathoracic structures must be considered in the light of a complete occupational history and the physical examination.

Physiologic changes in vascular patterns are due to several processes which influence the amount of blood present in arteries or veins or both at a given time. Some important influences are shunt effect, the phase of cardiac cycle, and the varying degrees of intrathoracic pressure present when the roentgenogram is recorded after the patient takes a deep breath and holds it.

When abnormal intrapulmonary changes develop, vessel shadows become less well defined. Increased prominence of vessel shadows under such circumstances occurs rarely, if at all.

Emphysema, as a rule, is not well portrayed in P-A roentgenograms of coal workers' pneumoconiosis. I have the impression that in the presence of well-established emphysema, the shadow pattern of preexisting small opacities may lose some or all of their identity (Fig. 22). By the same deduction, it is reasonable to anticipate that the shadow pattern of small opacities may not be seen in the presence of advanced generalized emphysema of a soft-coal worker who has a long history of dust exposure.

The patterns of small opacities found in the pneumoconiosis of soft-

Survey		Rounded Small Opacities			Irregular Small Opacities			Large Opacities		Pleural Thickening					Ill-Defined Diaphragm	Ill-Defined Cardiac Outline	Pleural Calcification					Reader ____ Date ____	
Number (1)	Quality (2)	Type (3)	Profusion (4)	Zones R L (5)	Type (6)	Profusion (7)	Zones R L (8)	Type (9)	Size (10)	Costophrenic angle (11)	Diffuse (12)	Plaques (13)	Grade (14)	None (15)	(16)	(17)	Diaphragm (18)	Wall (19)	Others (20)	Grade (21)	None (22)	Symbols (23)	Comment (24)
		p	0/- 0/0 0/1		s	0/- 0/0 0/1		wd	O A	O R L	R L		0 1 2 3	O if none	O R L	O 1 2		R L		0 1 2 3	O if none	O ca es co od cp tba	
	+	q	1/0 1/1 1/2		t	1/0 1/1 1/2		id	B														
	±	r	2/1 2/2 2/3		u	2/1 2/2 2/3			C														
	= U/R		3/2 3/3 3/4			3/2 3/3 3/4																	

FIG. 17. Recording sheet for classification of radiographic appearances of pneumoconiosis, without notations. In epidemiologic studies, it is extremely important that at least one entry must be made between each pair of heavy lines. When one is recording a single study, some modification is necessary if the large form seems inappropriate.

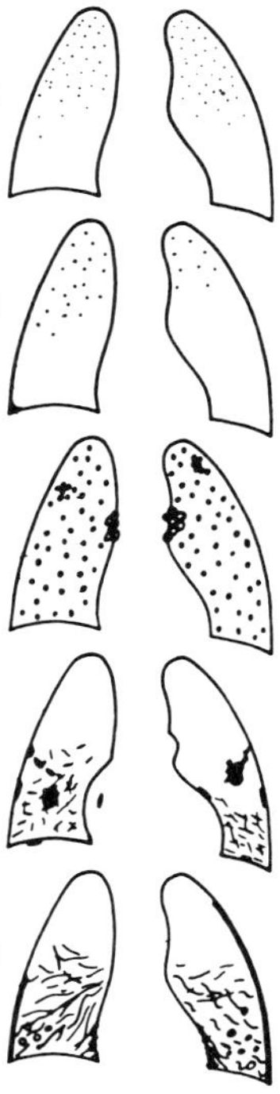

Number	Quality	Rounded small opacities: Type	Rounded small opacities: Profusion	Rounded small opacities: Zones (R L)	Irregular small opacities: Type	Irregular small opacities: Profusion	Irregular small opacities: Zones (R L)	Large opacities: Type	Large opacities: Size	Castophrenic angle	Pleural thickening: Diffuse	Pleural thickening: Plaques	Pleural thickening: Grade	Pleural thickening: None	Ill defined diaphragm	Ill defined cardiac outline	Pleural calcification: Diaphragm	Pleural calcification: Wall	Pleural calcification: Other	Pleural calcification: Grade	Pleural calcification: None	Symbols	Comments
1		p	2/2	✓✓ / ✓✓ / ––		0/0			0	0				0	0	0					0	0	0
2		q	1/2	✓✓ / ✓– / ––		0/0			0	R				0	0	0					0	0	0
3		r	3/3	✓✓ / ✓✓ / ✓✓		0/0			0	0				0	0	0					0	es ax	0
4			0/0		s	2/1	✓– / –– / ✓✓		0	0				0	0	0	L R	L R	L R	3		cp	Calcified plaque on pericardium
5			0/0		t	3/2	–– / ✓✓ / ✓✓		0	0	L F		3		0	2					0	ho	0
6			0/0		u	2/1	–– / –– / ✓✓		0	0		L	1		0	0					0	ca	ca = Mesotheliome
7		q	2/2	✓✓ / ✓✓ / ––		0/0		wd	B	0				0	0	0					0	bu	0
8			0/0		t	3/4	✓✓ / ✓✓ / ✓✓	id	B	L R	L R		1		L R	3					0	0	0
9		r	1/0	✓✓ / ✓✓ / ––		0/0			0	L R				0	0	0					0	di tba cv	? Silico-tuberculosis
10		p	2/1	✓✓ / ✓✓ / ––	s	2/3	✓– / ✓✓ / ✓✓		0	0				0	0	0					0	ca k	0
	+ ± ‡ U/R	p q r	0/– 0/0 0/1 1/0 1/1 1/2 2/1 2/2 2/3 3/2 3/3 3/4	Check zones involved	s t u	0/– 0/0 0/1 1/0 1/1 1/2 2/1 2/2 2/3 3/2 3/3 3/4	Check zones involved	wd id	0 A B C	0 R L	R L		1 2 3	0 If none	0 R L	0 1 2 3	R L			1 2 3	0 If none	0 ca es co od cp tba	

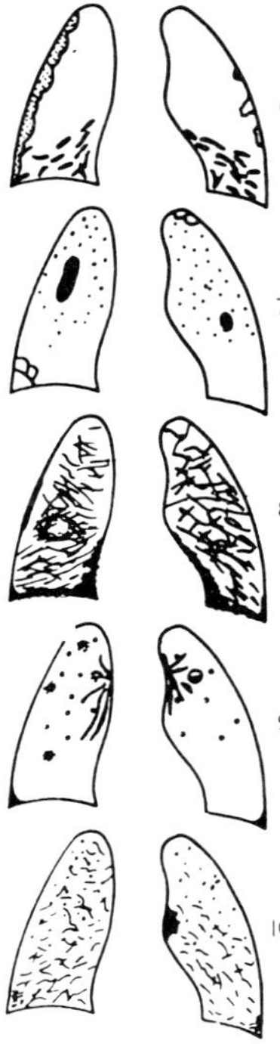

FIG. 18. Schematic representation of some radiographic featu:es. Compare the pattern illustrated in the chest diagrams with the numbers and symbols recorded on the report form.

coal miners of Pennsylvania are similar to those which occur in anthracosilicosis and graphite workers' pneumoconiosis (16, 17). However, in
many instances the opacities are largely in the lower half of the lung
field, whereas in anthracite miners of Pennsylvania, they more often are
seen in the upper two-thirds of the lung fields. The abnormal changes
include micronodular densities, lace-like and sponge-like shadows, Kerley
lines, and pleural thickening and calcification [Figs. 3, 15(A), and 15(B)].
The pattern of changes not infrequently simulates the appearance of a
moderately advanced asbestosis (18).

Large opacities vary in size from 3–15 cm or more. They may be single
or multiple, round, elongated, triangular, or oval in shape. They occur
in the upper, middle, or lower lung fields on one or both sides. A single
massive lesion may extend to the interlobar fissure, or if two are present,
one on either side of the fissure, they may grow toward each other and
obliterate the fissure. On the roentgenogram the lesions ultimately appear
as a single mass.

Large opacities may be located anteriorly or posteriorly and may occur
in the mid or peripheral, or both, portions of the lobe. It is necessary to
make P-A, lateral, and oblique views to determine their exact position
(Figs. 20 and 21).

Massive lesions, when present, sometimes are caused by undrained
cavities or cysts filled with black fluid (Fig. 19). The cavities and cysts
may appear on the roentgenograms as either massive lesions or cavities
with or without fluid levels, depending on whether or not there is communication with a bronchus. If cysts and cavities contain air, they may be
thick- or thin-walled, regular or irregular.

Cavities and cysts are thought to be due to liquefaction necrosis from
infection (19), carcinoma of the lung with central necrosis, or ischemic
necrosis (20). In necrosis due to carcinoma, the walls are usually thick
and irregular.

Theodos et al. (21), in a study of 1980 anthracite-coal miners during a
13-year period, made the following interesting observations on large
opacities: When conglomerate masses were asymmetrical, generally, an
associated infection was found; definite cavities were seen in the roentgenogram of 206 or 10.4% of the 1980 coal miners.

If a positive sputum could not be obtained in the presence of cavitation,
then neoplasm, lung abscess, and fungus disease had to be excluded. If
none of them were found, cavitation was attributed to ischemic necrosis.

In 206 cases with cavitation, acid-fast bacilli were found by smear or
culture in 141, or 68.4%. Carcinoma of the lung accounted for two cases
of cavitation; cystic bronchiectasis for two; and no adequate cause of
cavitation could be ascertained in four cases.

The remaining 57 cases, or 27% with cavitation, were attributed to ischemic necrosis. Cavitation appeared as a unilateral process in 37; it was bilateral in 19 instances. In 20 cases, the cavitation appeared initially as a large opacity; in 6 of the 20, the cavities were filled with secretions

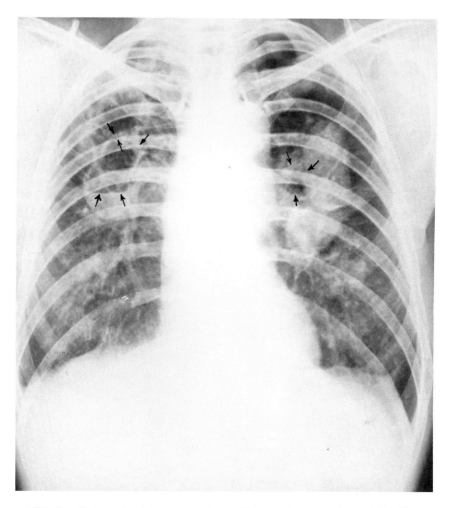

FIG. 19. Coal workers' pneumoconiosis with cysts in the right and left lungs. Note the thickness of the cavity walls and the air and fluid levels (arrows). These cysts are not thought to be due to an infection such as tubercle, staphylococcus, or Friedlanders bacillus. They are thought to be due to necrosis resulting from anemia infarcts. The cysts may fill and the evidence of the cavity then will disappear. They do not have the symptoms and signs of an active infection. These cysts may be small or large. In addition to the large opacities which may represent infarcts that do not communicate with a bronchus, there are many small irregular opacities *u*. There is some peaking of the domes of the diaphragm due to inelasticity of the lungs.

and were invisible. The cavities were small, slit-like, or large. Their contents were ink-like, nonpurulent, and of a maple-syrup-like consistency.

The clinical picture of ischemic necrosis rarely included fever, toxicity, or generalized debility. A benign course of cavitation due to ischemia was readily distinguished from that due to tuberculosis. The ischemic process was followed as long as 11 years.

The authors emphasized the importance of recognizing the nontuberculous nature of the cavitation to avoid hospitalization in a tuberculous facility and permit the miner to live in normal relationship to his family and the community, as well as to be gainfully employed if pulmonary function permits.

When massive lesions and emphysema develop, the background pattern of small opacities may largely disappear (Fig. 22). It also seems important to be aware that the pattern of abnormal changes in coal workers' pneumoconiosis may vary from mine to mine in central and western Pennsylvania (4–8) and from state to state in the United States.

MASSIVE FIBROSIS AND CARCINOMA

Unilateral well-defined large opacities in coal miners may represent carcinoma, cyst, or massive fibrosis. There may or may not be a background of small opacities. The lesion may remain unchanged for 1–5 years. There may be a history of hemoptysis and a suspicious looking cytological smear.

Another type of massive lesion simulates a pattern of encroachment, fixation, and constriction of a large main bronchus. Such an appearance may occur in primary massive fibrosis or carcinoma. Operative removal may be the only way by which the lesion can be identified.

MIGRATION OF MASSIVE LESIONS

Massive lesions may migrate centrally. When such a massive lesion becomes part of the shadow complex of the mediastinum, the roentgenographic appearance simulates a tumor and has been so diagnosed and treated [Figs. 20(A)–20(D)].

Large opacities, seen in lateral views, may be anterior or posterior to the midline of the thorax. Major migration of large masses is a slow process. Such migration may require 5–25 years (Figs. 20 and 21).

Gough (22) noted that when massive fibrosis causes shrinkage of the upper portions of the lung, severe bullous emphysema may develop. On occasions, in bullous emphysema the shadow pattern simulates a large opacity due to the crowding and distortion effect of the adjacent lung parenchyma.

When tuberculosis without cavitation is present in massive lesions,

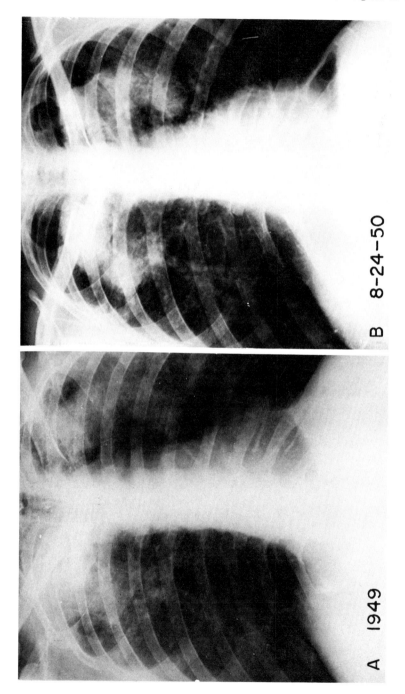

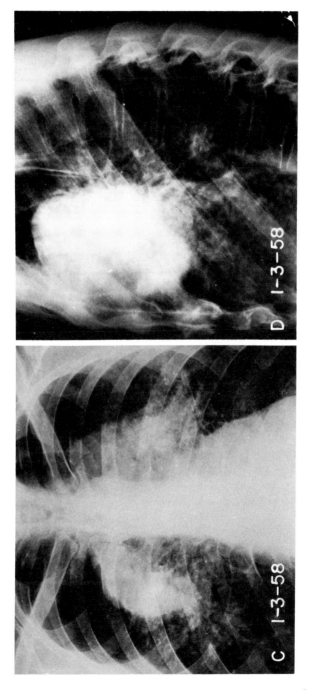

FIG. 20. Complicated coal workers' pneumoconiosis, category 2 r, C, em, hi, di, in which there is evidence of migration of large opacities. (A) 1949; (B) 1950, slight evidence of migration toward the midline; (C) 1958, further evidence of migration; (D) 1958, the two opacities have migrated anteriorly and appear as a single opacity in the lateral view.

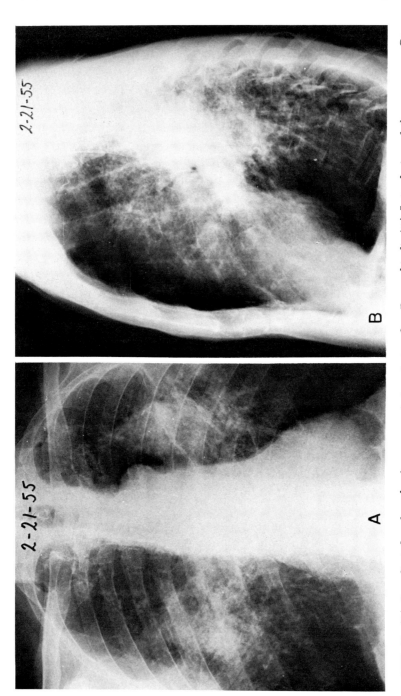

FIG. 21. (A) Complicated coal workers' pneumoconiosis, category 2 *r*, B, em, hi, di. (B) Lateral view of the same case. Compare with Fig. 20(D). In this instance the lesions have migrated posteriorly. In workers who have large opacities, lateral views sometimes provide important information.

multiple areas of calcification may be noted throughout the large opacity. At first, calcification within the large opacity is scarcely visible, but over the years the deposition of calcium becomes more prominent. It may also appear within lymph nodes. One cannot differentiate between the calcification of histoplasmosis and that of tuberculosis from the roentgenographic appearance. Tubercle bacilli are found in less than 50% of massive lesions (22). However, tuberculosis is so serious a complication that, from the radiologic standpoint, one should report massive lesions with or without cavity as suspicious of tuberculosis so that appropriate clinical and bacteriological studies can be carried out to diagnose or exclude a tuberculous process.

RHEUMATOID CHANGES

These changes were described by Caplan (23) in 1952. The roentgenographic lesions are round or irregularly round, well defined, 1–5 cm or larger in size, bilateral, often peripheral, and usually rapid in development (but once developed, they remain unchanged for years). There is usually a background of micronodulation of pneumoconiosis. Rheumatoid nodules may undergo liquefaction. Some show small areas of dense calcification (24).

Miall (25) described a similar pattern of lesions in the lung in patients with rheumatoid arthritis uncomplicated by coal workers' pneumoconiosis. He and others confirmed that inheritance is important in the etiology of the disease. Some rheumatoid changes simulate silicosis, sarcoidosis, and other conditions with patterns of widespread nodulation (26).

In one patient in which there was no history of harmful dust exposure, a single large opacity due to a rheumatoid granuloma was removed because of a presumptive diagnosis of carcinoma of the lung (27).

HEART DISEASE

It has long been known clinically that cor pulmonale was often the mode of death in the pneumoconiosis of coal miners: "Cor pulmonale is common in progressive massive fibrosis, but rare with simple pneumoconiosis. Severe vascular lesions are associated with the former but rarely with simple pneumoconiosis (1 [p. 16])."

Wells, in Gough's department and mentioned by Gough (22), studied the arterial tree at postmortem examination after injecting opaque material. The roentgen examination of the specimen shows considerable reduction in the pulmonary tree, due to the various forms of arterial obstruction such as endarteritis, thrombosis, massive fibrosis, and emphysema. Cor pulmonale was present often. "The presence of such vascular changes is not necessarily the major cause of cor pulmonale (1 [p. 16])."

From a group of 375 hard-coal miners with various categories of anthracosilicosis, electrocardiograms were done on 148 patients. The reasons for the choice of those 148 patients were not given. Of those, 24 or 16.2% showed evidence of strain of the right side of the heart (28). There appeared to be no correlation between stage of anthracosilicosis as determined by the roentgenogram and incidence of strain of the right side of the heart.

Cor pulmonale with increased preponderance in the size of the right side of the heart is difficult to evaluate on a single chest roentgenogram. If serial roentgenograms with P-A, oblique, and lateral views are available, one may observe an increased preponderance in the size of the right heart.

The conventional roentgenogram of the chest for cardiac disease is not very revealing in the presence of large and small opacities and emphysema. The vascular pattern of pulmonary vessels cannot be evaluated, because it may be obscured by the small opacities. The size and shape of the heart may not be informative because of distortion due to the lung lesions.

PLEURAL ABNORMALITIES

Involvement of the pleura in coal workers' pneumoconiosis is not as dominant as in asbestosis, but it does occur, and it is important that the abnormalities be recorded.

Pleural thickening may manifest itself as pleural plaques, generalized thickening, and obliteration of the costophrenic sulci (Fig. 13). Such changes may involve the domes of the diaphragm, the interlobar pleura, the walls of the thorax, and the cardiac pleura. Slight pleural thickening on the anterior and posterior walls and in interlobar fissures are seen in oblique and lateral projections, but may not be in P-A and A-P projections. We do not attempt to record pleural "caps." Slight and even definite costophrenic obliteration and interlobar thickening may result from preexisting inflammatory processes. This is always considered in our evaluation.

The pleural thickening may be generalized or occur as plaques. So-called "peaking" of the domes of the diaphragm is a form of pleural thickening especially at the sites of the interlobar fissures, but one should be mindful that a similar pattern may be produced in inspiration by an "inelasticity" of the adjacent intralobar bronchial and vascular structures and other tissues (Fig. 22).

Pleural calcification occurs either as plaques or in generalized forms in coal workers who do not have a positive history of exposure to asbestos dust (7, 8). Plaques are easily overlooked when they occur on areas of the domes of the diaphragm or chest walls that are not recorded in an axial view.

Pneumothorax is seen occasionally in coal workers' pneumoconiosis and is easily recognized (Fig. 23).

Pleural collections oftentimes are observed in cardiac decompensation or as a complication to some pulmonary infection or malignancy.

CONCLUSION AND SUMMARY

In conclusion, it seems important and appropriate to again emphasize a few observations that have been recorded elsewhere. They are:

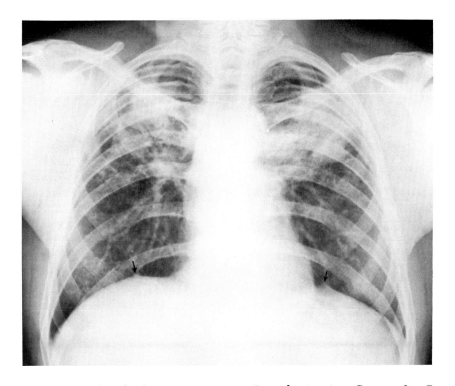

FIG. 22. Coal workers' pneumoconiosis in a Pennsylvania miner, Category 2 *q*, B, em, hi, di. The small opacities are largely obscured by the large opacities and the emphysema. The hila are displaced upward, and one can see the stretch effect due to distortion and the upward pull on the hila and the pulmonary vessels. Note the peaking of the domes of the diaphragm (arrows).

Coal workers' pneumoconiosis cannot be diagnosed in the living in the absence of radiographic changes. There is no characteristic physiological derangement which is indicative of dust in the lungs (1 [p. 25]).

The most desirable chest radiograph for the study of pneumoconiosis or other pulmonary disease is one in which the lung is shown in greatest detail (1 [p. 27]).

The conventional chest roentgenogram has no value in establishing the presence or severity of chronic bronchitis (1 [pp. 31–33]).

A mechanism should be developed for distribution in the United States of standard ILO films to any interested physician, radiology department, or investigator in pneumoconiosis (1 [p. 32]), and all men in the coal

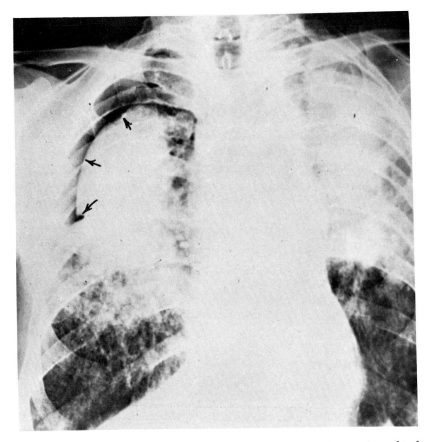

FIG. 23. Complicated coal workers' pneumoconiosis, category 2 *r*, *u*, C pn, hi, di, with a pneumothorax on the right. Note that there is no visible pattern of adhesions modifying a partial collapse of the right upper lobe.

industry should have a preemployment medical examination including chest radiographs and pulmonary function studies. These examinations should be repeated at least at 5-year intervals.* This material should be collected in a manner suitable for scientific examination as well as clinical use (1 [p. 32]).

Prospective studies of the natural history of coal workers' pneumoconiosis are needed, and they should be correlated with all environmental factors. One goal of these studies should be to determine the relationship between the exposure and the risk of disease, resulting in a determination of guidelines for permissible safe exposure for the miners' working lifetime (1 [pp. 32–33]).

Proper correlation of pathological findings with clinical, X-ray, and physiological studies have been seriously impaired by the lack of autopsy material. Effective mechanisms must be developed which will provide access to autopsy material in conjunction with other studies. An adequate central facility should be available for the study of that material (1 [p. 33]).

This chapter includes critical comments on the essentials of chest radiography as it concerns equipment and technique; roentgenographic patterns of coal workers' pneumoconiosis in the United States; the aims, principles, and details of the U/C Classification of the radiographic appearances of pneumoconioses; and the radiologic considerations of the interpretation and evaluation of the shadow patterns as they obtain to the occupational history and the physical examination.

REFERENCES

1. International Conference on C.W.P. (1969). "Synopsis of the Work Session Proceedings," Sept. 10–12. Spindletop Res., Inc., Lexington, Ky.
2. Pendergrass, E. P. (1970). *Arch. Environ. Health* **20**, 545.
3. Jacobson, G., Bohlig, H., and Kiviluoto, R. (1970). *Radiology* **95**, 445.
4. Lainhart, W. S. (1969). *J. Occup. Med.* **11**, 399.
5. Lieben, J., Pendergrass, E. P., and McBride, W. W. (1961). *J. Occup. Med.* **3**, 493.
6. McBride, W. W., Pendergrass, E. P., and Lieben, J. (1963). *J. Occup. Med.* **5**, 376.
7. Lieben, J., and McBride, W. W. (1963). *J. Amer. Med. Ass.* **183**, 176.
8. Baier, E. J., and Diakun, R. (1961). *J. Occup. Med.* **3**, 507.
9. "A Cooperative Study: Radiologic Classification of the Pneumoconioses" (1966). *Arch. Environ. Health* **12**, 314.
10. Gilson, J. C., *et al.* (1970). *Chest* **58**, 57.
11. Liddell, F. D. K. (1963). *Brit. J. Ind. Med.* **20**, 300.

* The Federal Coal Mine Health and Safety Act of 1969 substantially makes these requirements.

12. Liddell, F. D. K., and May, J. A. (1966). "Assessing the Radiological Progression of Simple Pneumoconiosis," *Nat. Coal Board Med. Res. Memo.* 4. Hobart House, London.
13. Rae, S. (1971). "The Reduction of Observer Variation in Categorizing Coal Workers' Pneumoconiosis." *Proc. Int. Conf. Pneumoconiosis, Johannesburg, 1969.* (In Press).
14. Gilson, J. C., Davies, T. A. L., and Oldham, P. D. "A Study of Respiratory Responses to Duration of Foundry Work." *Proc. Int. Conf. Pneumonconiosis, Johannesburg, 1969.* (In press.)
15. Weber, A. L., *et al.* (1966). "Roentgen Manifestations of Asbestosis," *Int. Congr. Occup. Health, Vienna, 1966.*
16. Pendergrass, E. P., *et al.* (1967). *Med. Radiog. Photog.* **43**, 69.
17. Pendergrass, E. P., *et al.* (1968). *Med. Radiog. Photog.* **44**, 1.
18. Pendergrass, E. P., Lieben, J., and McBride, W. W. (1963). *Excerpta Med. Found.* 3, 1152.
19. Wall, N. M. (1955). *Amer. Rev. Tuberc. Pulm. Dis.* **71**, 344.
20. Vorwald, A. J. (1941). *Amer. J. Pathol.* **17**, 709.
21. Theodos, P. A., Cathcart, R. T., and Fraimow, W. (1961). *Arch. Environ. Health* **2**, 609.
22. Gough, J. (1952). "Patterns in Pneumoconiosis," *Fourth Conf. McIntyre Res. Found. Silicosis, Noranda, Quebec.*
23. Caplan, A. (1953). *Thorax* **8**, 29.
24. Gough, J., Rivers, D., and Seal, R. M. E. (1955). *Thorax* **10**, 9.
25. Miall, W. E. (1955). *Ann. Rheum. Dis.* **14**, 150.
26. Price, T. M. L., and Skelton, M. O. (1956). *Thorax* **11**, 234.
27. Collins, L. H., Margolies, M., and Pendergrass, E. P. (1969). *Pa. Med.* **72**, 53.
28. Theodos, P. A., Gordon, B., and Lang, L. P. (1950). *Dis. Chest.* **17**, 249.

8

Pulmonary Function

N. LeRoy Lapp and Anthony Seaton

The pulmonary function abnormalities found among coal workers depend to a large extent upon the population studied. Most reports in the United States literature are of studies of symptomatic subjects, but several investigations of random samples of miners and exminers have been published. The results in the two types of study differ, but even in the random samples there probably exists an element of selection in that the less fit may migrate from the industry. The extent of this migration and the factors that influence it are at present unknown.

The findings presented in this report represent a summary of the current knowledge of abnormalities of pulmonary function associated with coal workers' pneumoconiosis. For convenience the pulmonary functional abnormalities have been grouped under the headings of ventilatory capacity, mechanics, diffusion, gas exchange, and pulmonary hemodynamics. In keeping with the selection bias mentioned above, the functional abnormalities have been discussed in the light of whether they have been found in symptomatic, asymptomatic, or randomly chosen subjects. A list of abbreviations used throughout this book is given in Table I. The classification of radiographs in the text is that of the International Labour Organisation (1), except where otherwise stated (see Chapter 3, Fig. 1).

Ventilatory Capacity

We have been unable to find any studies of the pulmonary functional capacity of coal workers in the United States prior to 1949. In that year, Motley and co-workers (2) reported the results obtained from 100 symp-

TABLE I

ABBREVIATIONS USED IN TEXT OF BOOK

Proper names	
ALFORD	Appalachian Laboratory for Occupational Respiratory Diseases
CWP	Coal workers' pneumoconiosis
ILO	International Labour Organisation
MRE	Mining Research Establishment of (U. K.) National Coal Board
PMF	Progressive massive fibrosis
UICC	Union Internationale Contre le Cancer
Measures	
$(A-a)O_2$	Oxygen gradient between alveolar gas and arterial blood
D_L	Diffusing capacity of lung for carbon monoxide
FEV_1	Forced expiratory volume in 1 second
$FEV_{0.75}$	Forced expiratory volume in 0.75 or $\frac{3}{4}$ second
$FEF_{75\%}$	Expiratory flow at 75 % of forced vital capacity
$FEF_{25\%}$	Expiratory flow at 25 % of forced vital capacity
FRC	Functional residual capacity
FVC	Forced vital capacity
MBC	Maximal breathing capacity
MVV	Maximal voluntary ventilation
P_a	Arterial partial pressure
RV	Residual volume
TLC	Total lung capacity
VC	Vital capacity
V_D	Respiratory dead space
V_T	Tidal volume
Radiographic	
P-A	Posteroanterior direction of beam
A-P	Anteroposterior direction of beam

tomatic anthracite miners between the ages of 40 and 65 years. All but one of these subjects complained of dyspnea, and all had long histories of underground exposure. All subjects had radiographic evidence of pneumoconiosis of varying degrees. The parameters studied were vital capacity (VC), maximal voluntary ventilation (MVV), residual volume (RV), and total lung capacity (TLC). The subjects were classified according to the RV/TLC ratio into groups with normal function, slight, moderate, advanced, and far-advanced emphysema. The investigators were unable to demonstrate significant correlations between the ventilatory abnormalities and either length of exposure to mine dust or stage of radiographic abnormality.

A similar study of 56 symptomatic bituminous-coal miners was conducted by Motley and associates (3). The miners were selected largely from clinics in the Appalachian states. The findings in this group were similar to those observed among anthracite miners, namely, that all degrees of emphysema (increased RV/TLC ratio) were found in all age groups and there was a poor correlation between functional and radiographic abnormalities and of the duration of exposure to mine dust.

In a study of a group of 242 working miners aged 45–65 years from Pennsylvania, Ohio, and West Virginia, Pemberton (4) utilized the forced expiratory volume in 1 second (FEV₁) as an index of ventilatory capacity. He also studied comparable groups of workers in two factories, one located in an urban area, the other located in a rural area. When considered as a group, a higher proportion of the coal miners had an FEV₁ that was less than 65% of predicted normal than did either factory group. This difference was most notable among subjects older than age 55 and was observed despite the fact that the average cigarette consumption among the two factory groups was greater than in the coal miner group. Neither a significantly greater number of symptoms nor a greater decrease in FEV₁ were observed among the working miners with radiographic evidence of pneumoconiosis than among those without pneumoconiosis.

In a study comparing symptomatic miners who had worked mainly as handloaders to those who had been predominantly motormen, Anderson and co-workers (5) found a significant excess of radiographic lesions greater than 3 mm in diameter among the motormen. The handloaders showed an excess of lesions less than 3 mm in diameter. In this group of 153 handloaders and 53 motormen, no striking differences were demonstrated between the two categories with regard to symptoms of exertional dyspnea, although a slightly greater number of motormen had an MVV of less than 60% of predicted normal.

Hyatt and co-workers (6) studied a random sample of 167 bituminous-coal miners and exminers, 45–58 years old, in a geographic unit in southern West Virginia. The sample was stratified according to the number of years worked underground. The prevalence of simple pneumoconiosis was 39%, while a further 7% had the complicated form of the disease. While the severity of pneumoconiosis was related to the number of years worked underground, there was no apparent relation to the number of years worked at the coal face as opposed to the total number of years spent underground.

These authors utilized the FEF₂₅₋₇₅% as a measurement of ventilatory capacity, but they also measured FEV₁, VC, TLC, and RV/TLC ratio. They found increasing impairment of ventilatory function and increasing symptoms with increasing duration of underground work. Only in category-3*-simple and complicated diseases, however, could it be demonstrated that pneumoconiosis impaired ventilatory function. The interrelations of symptoms to duration of underground work, pulmonary

* For significance of categories, see Chapter 3, p. 32 and Fig. 1.

function, and presence and severity of pneumoconiosis were not simple. A definite association between years worked underground and impairment of pulmonary function was found, which was not adequately explained by age, smoking habits, or category of pneumoconiosis.

Higgins and associates (7) studied 425 miners and exminers, and 399 nonminers in five mining communities in northern West Virginia. All males between the ages of 20 and 69 living in three towns were invited to be examined, and 83% responded. The ventilatory test that was used to assess functional status was the FEV_1. This study showed that FEV_1 was significantly decreased in miners and exminers with 30 years or more of underground experience. In those who had less than 30 years exposure underground the FEV_1 of miners and exminers was not significantly different from the FEV_1 of nonminers from the same communities. No apparent effect of cigarette smoking upon ventilatory function was evident in these subjects until age 50. In the two oldest age groups, 50–59 and 60–69, cigarette smokers and exsmokers recorded a lower mean FEV_1 than nonsmokers.

Rasmussen and co-workers (8) reported the results of studies of 192 symptomatic miners from southern West Virginia. Approximately 40% of these men were working in the mines at the time of the study, and of those who were unemployed at the time, 75% had left because of an inability to continue working. These workers were unable to find a correlation between advancing radiographic category and ventilatory impairment in their subjects. Further, using the indices of FEV_1, $FEF_{25-75\%}$, TLC, and RV/TLC ratio, they were unable to demonstrate any definite relationship between ventilatory impairment and other factors such as age, years in the industry, or cigarette smoking.

Henschel (9) recently reported the results of a U. S. Public Health Service study of a sample of 2432 working miners and 1028 nonworking miners (the nonworking miners were not working for reasons of health, age, or unemployment, or they were working at jobs other than coal mining) from the Appalachian bituminous-coal mining areas. The FVC in this group of miners decreased with increasing age but was little different from the predicted value for normal subjects of comparable age. On the other hand, the FEV_1 was lower than predicted in the older subjects than could be accounted for by aging alone. The average decrease in observed FEV_1 from the predicted value was from 6–9% in the working miners and from 12–20% in the nonworking miners.

When the ventilatory function of these subjects was expressed as the ratio of FEV_1/FVC, a consistent decline with advancing age was noted, but only in the two older age groups (40–50 and over 50 years) of nonworking miners was this value less than 70%. This decrease in FEV_1 with a normal FVC indicates some degree of airflow obstruction, particularly among the older nonworking miners. It may also indicate some tendency for migration of the less fit from mining, leaving a selected population among the working miners.

A definite effect of cigarette smoking upon ventilatory function was observed in this study. Cigarette smokers in both the working and nonworking groups had a lower FEV_1 than nonsmokers, but there was no clear linear decrease with increasing number of cigarettes smoked per day.

A slight decrease in FVC with increasing number of years spent underground, not accounted for by increasing age, was noted among working miners. The FEV_1 in working miners decreased with increasing number of years spent underground but to a greater extent than did the FVC. This finding suggests a relationship between airflow obstruction and duration of underground exposure that cannot be attributed to age alone. Among the nonworking miners, no clear relationship between declining ventilatory function, as measured by the FEV_1/FVC ratio, and number of years spent underground was observed.

Of all the comparisons made between clinical findings, symptoms, and ventilatory function, dyspnea was most closely correlated with alterations in the FVC and FEV_1. In both the working and nonworking miners, the ratio of FEV_1/FVC declined with increasing degree of dyspnea, as did the ratio of the observed to predicted FEV_1. The relationship between pulmonary functional status and a history of bronchitis was less obvious. In general, there was a decrease in FEV_1 and the ratio of FEV_1/FVC in those working miners who reported episodes of bronchitis as compared to those who reported none. However, no differences in ventilatory function could be demonstrated between those working miners who were classified as having "simple" bronchitis and those having "multiple" episodes of bronchitis.

When ventilatory capacity of working miners was compared with radiographic category of pneumoconiosis, it was shown that FVC was not appreciably altered with increasing lung involvement. The FEV_1, however, was lower than the predicted value in those working miners with no radiographic evidence of pneumoconiosis and declined further in those with simple pneumoconiosis. A slight further decrease in FEV_1 was seen in those working miners with complicated pneumoconiosis.

Recently, the residual volume (RV) and total capacity (TLC) of 705 working Pennsylvania coal miners were determined as part of a larger epidemiological study undertaken by personnel of the Appalachian Laboratory for Occupational Respiratory Diseases (10). The effect of increasing radiographic category of pneumoconiosis on lung volumes was investigated. The results were expressed as the mean ratio of observed to predicted RV and related to the radiographic category of pneumoconiosis. It was shown that the RV increased with radiographic category and that this occurred whether or not the miners had obstructive airway disease as defined by an FEV_1/FVC ratio of greater or less than 70%. A larger increase in RV was found in those miners who had both obstruction (FEV_1/FVC less than 70%) and radiographic evidence of pneumoconiosis than in those who had no obstruction (FEV_1/FVC greater than 70%) but who had pneumoconiosis (Figs. 1 and 2). The mean TLC of miners in this study was somewhat lower than the predicted value, but when expressed as the ratio of observed to predicted TLC and compared to radiographic category, no relationship was observed.

In summary, the ventilatory capacity of working and nonworking miners is generally lower than the predicted normal. In those with symptoms, a decrease in ventilatory capacity correlates best with smoking

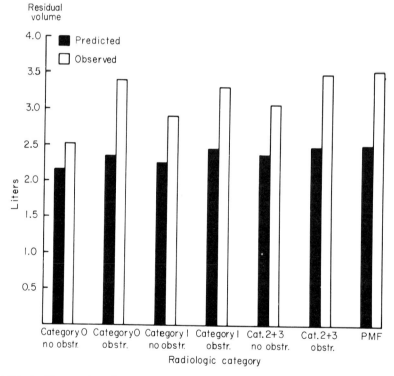

FIG. 1. The predicted and observed mean residual volume (BTPS) for seven groups of working miners with and without obstruction in relation to radiographic category of pneumoconiosis.

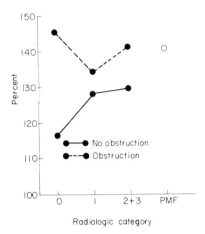

FIG. 2. The ratio of observed to predicted residual volume expressed as a percentage plotted versus radiographic category of pneumoconiosis for working miners with and without obstruction. The marked increase in the ratio of observed to predicted among subjects with category 0 and obstruction is due to the small number of subjects, many of whom have asthma.

habits, and there is poor correlation between ventilatory capacity and both duration of dust exposure and radiographic category. Ventilatory capacity is also reduced in working miners, especially in those over 50 years of age, and in general the decrease correlates with duration of dust exposure and radiographic category of pneumoconiosis. Cigarette smoking appears to exert an added effect of decreasing ventilatory function in working miners.

Mechanics

Leathart (11) investigated pulmonary mechanics in 97 British coal workers, many of whom were disabled or claiming compensation. He found a slight decrease in compliance with increasing age and time spent underground, but this was not significantly related to radiographic category. Inspiratory airway resistance was normal in all subjects, but the nonelastic work of respiration was increased in many, presumably due to expiratory airway obstruction. Ferris and Frank (12) reported an investigation of 25 Appalachian soft-coal miners, all of whom were symptomatic. Two of these subjects, both with complicated pneumoconiosis, had reduced lung compliance. The change in dynamic compliance at different rates of respiration was investigated in a few of these subjects. In those with normal pulmonary resistance there was, as in elderly normal subjects, little fall in compliance at increased respiratory rates. In those

TABLE II

MECHANICS IN SUBJECTS WITH SIMPLE CWP

Group	Number of patients		Age (years)	C stat[a] (liter/cm H₂O)	C dyn[b] (liter/cm H₂O)	Pel[c] (cm H₂O)	$\frac{\text{C stat}}{\text{FRC}}$	$\frac{\text{C dyn}}{\text{C stat}}$	$\frac{\text{P}_{\text{el}}}{\text{TLC}}$
0	22	Mean	52.1	0.231	0.198	24.6	0.056	0.799	4.1
		S.D.	(10.5)	(0.152)	(0.107)	(15.1)	(0.032)	(0.316)	(1.8)
1	24	Mean	58.5	0.252	0.163	26.7	0.062	0.697	4.2
		S.D.	(7.3)	(0.105)	(0.072)	(7.9)	(0.025)	(0.222)	(1.3)
2	15	Mean	54.7	0.242	0.172	29.4	0.073	0.750	4.8
		S.D.	(6.8)	(0.150)	(0.093)	(13.7)	(0.046)	(0.336)	(2.3)
3	5	Mean	52.6	0.257	0.188	20.5	0.052	0.833	3.9
		S.D.	(7.4)	(0.193)	(0.098)	(12.1)	(0.022)	(0.315)	(1.2)
Normal Range				0.18–0.28	0.13–0.28	23–37	0.07–0.04	> 0.8	3.5–7.5

[a] Static compliance.
[b] Dynamic compliance.
[c] Pulmonary recoil pressure at TLC.

with increased airway resistance, compliance fell as the rate of respiration increased. In addition, these authors found pulmonary flow resistance to be increased significantly in the group of subjects with most disability as compared to that in those with least disability. They were, however, unable to find any consistent differences in static recoil pressure at TLC between their patients, whether grouped according to disability or to radiographic category.

In order to study the effects on pulmonary mechanics of coal workers' pneumoconiosis uncomplicated by obstructive airway disease, 66 symptomatic but unobstructed coal workers were studied at the Appalachian Laboratory for Occupational Respiratory Diseases. All had an FEV_1/FVC of 70% or greater. They were divided into groups according to their radiographic category, as follows:

Group 0—22 subjects with no radiographic evidence of CWP
Group 1—24 subjects with category 1 CWP
Group 2—15 subjects with category 2 CWP
Group 3—5 subjects with either category 3 or complicated CWP (stage A)

In most of these subjects, static and dynamic compliance and pulmonary recoil pressures at TLC and FRC were studied. The results (Table II) show that the mean values for most indices measured in all groups fell within the normal range.

In each group a few individuals fell outside the normal range. This is illustrated by examining the coefficient of retraction in these subjects, as suggested by Schleuter and co-workers (13). These results are recorded in Table III. The normal range for this measurement (pulmonary elastic pressure at TLC divided by TLC) is taken to be 3.5–7.5 cm of water/liter of TLC. Emphysematous subjects have values below 3.5, while those with pulmonary fibrosis show values greater than 7.5. Thus, of these 63 subjects, 22 had low coefficients of retraction, while only three had high

TABLE III
Coefficient of Retraction in Unobstructed Coal Workers

	Number of subjects with:		
Group	Normal coefficient	Low coefficient	High coefficient
0	13	7	1
1	14	9	0
2	7	5	2
3	4	1	0

TABLE IV

MECHANICS IN SUBJECTS WITH COMPLICATED CWP

Radio-graphic category	Number of subjects	Age (years)	$\dfrac{\text{FEV}_1}{\text{FVC}}$	C stat (liter/cm H_2O)	C dyn (liter/cm H_2O)	P_{el} at TLC (cm H_2O)	$\dfrac{\text{C dyn}}{\text{C stat}}$	P_{el}/TLC (cm H_2O/liter)
B	16	Mean 65.2	55.5	0.210	0.143	32.2	0.777	4.9
		S.D. (8.5)	(16.2)	(0.104)	(0.060)	(15.6)	(0.391)	(2.3)
C	9	Mean 56.7	62.4	0.158	0.095	32.8	0.666	5.8
		S.D. (8.3)	(10.6)	(0.088)	(0.052)	(12.8)	(0.290)	(2.7)

coefficients. It seems, therefore, that symptomatic but unobstructed coal workers, with or without radiographic evidence of simple pneumoconiosis, either have normal pulmonary mechanics or less frequently have a low coefficient of retraction such as occurs in emphysema.

The ratio of dynamic to static compliance, obtained from the expiratory limb of the pressure–volume curve, tended to be at the lower limit of the normal range in these subjects. This difference could be accounted for by frequency dependence of this measurement in subjects with airway obstruction in the small peripheral airways (14, 15). Further studies are necessary to elucidate this point.

In addition, 16 symptomatic subjects with stage B and 9 with stage C complicated coal workers' pneumoconiosis have been studied at the Appalachian Laboratory. The mean results are recorded in Table IV, and the numbers of subjects with abnormal coefficients of retraction are shown in Table V. Again, the ratio of dynamic to static compliance is low, but in these cases obstruction in the main airways was frequently present and would account for this abnormality. In the stage B subjects, the coefficient of retraction was usually either normal or suggestive of emphysema, but in those with stage C disease there were more with a raised coefficient. It is likely that in subjects with complicated pneumoconiosis there is a balance between the opposing effects of fibrosis and compensatory overdistension, the effect of the former only showing itself when the lesions are very extensive.

TABLE V

COEFFICIENT OF RETRACTION IN SUBJECTS WITH COMPLICATED CWP

Category	Number of subjects with:		
	Normal coefficient	Low coefficient	High coefficient
B	9	5	2
C	3	2	4

In summary, the pulmonary mechanics in unobstructed miners with simple pneumoconiosis are usually normal. Deviation from the normal, when it occurs, is usually in the direction of an increase in compliance, when related to TLC, suggesting the presence of emphysema. In complicated pneumoconiosis more subjects may be found with a decreased compliance, especially in stage C, though again, increases are not uncommon, presumably a consequence of associated compensatory emphysema. There is some evidence that dynamic compliance in unobstructed coal workers may be frequency dependent, suggesting the presence of small airway disease.

Diffusion

There has been relatively little work reported in this field in the American and British literature. Gilson and Hugh-Jones (16) studied carbon monoxide uptake in a group of South Wales coal miners and found this to be slightly reduced in the older men and significantly decreased (by about 30%) in those with extensive complicated pneumoconiosis. Gaensler (17) reported a group of patients, two of whom were American coal miners, in whom a reduced single breath and steady-state diffusing capacity (D_L) was related to proven interstitial fibrosis and silicosis. Sartorelli et al. (18) studied 31 "silicotics" by the steady-state method and found the mean D_L to be at the lower end of the normal range. In general, those with pinpoint opacities (p) on the radiograph had a lower D_L than those with micronodular (m) lesions. Billiet (19), using the single-breath technique, studied 76 subjects with "anthracosilicosis" and found a progressive though slight diminution in D_L from radiographic category 0 or 1, through categories 2, 3, or A to B and C. Although the reduction in D_L was roughly proportional to the radiographic category, this was subject to a great deal of variation in individual subjects. Englert and DeCoster (20) studied single-breath D_L in 41 miners, using their own formulas for predicting normal results. They found subjects with category 0 or Z had normal D_L. Those subjects with the radiographic lesions of simple pneumoconiosis had slightly lower than normal values. Pinpoint radiographic opacities (p) were associated with a lower D_L on average than micronodular lesions (m). In subjects with m lesions, D_L divided by total lung capacity was normal, whereas in those with p lesions it tended to be reduced.

Vanroux and Gregoire (21) studied a series of men with micronodular pneumoconiosis by the steady-state method comparing the results with those from a large series of normal subjects. They found that in the miners, D_L did not increase to the expected degree on exertion and that

D_L divided by tidal volume decreased at higher levels of exercise, whereas in the normals this had remained fairly constant at 1.5.

Lavenne and co-workers (22) discussed the syndrome of alveolar–capillary block in Belgium coal workers' pneumoconiosis. On the basis of their physiologic and pathologic studies, they regarded the syndrome as uncommon. In the few cases in which they had encountered a low D_L they considered it to be due to ventilation–perfusion abnormalities and pointed out that low arterial oxygen tensions in these subjects were usually corrected by exercise. Podlesch and his colleagues (23) found 15% of 85 nonobstructed simple "silicotics" had a slightly reduced steady-state D_L at rest. This reduction only occurred in those subjects with categories 2 and 3 pneumoconiosis. The effect of different types of radiographic opacity was not mentioned. On the other hand, Nicaise and co-workers (24) investigated single-breath D_L in six subjects with micronodular category 2 and 3 and one with category A on a background of micronodular 2 pneumoconiosis; they found four to have a low D_L at rest and only one to increase to the expected degree on exercise. These subjects included four with a high residual volume, but the data given do not make clear whether obstructive airway disease was present.

Ogilvie and colleagues (25) studied 17 coal miners of whom two had a low single-breath D_L. Both these subjects had severe airway obstruction in addition to their pneumoconiosis. Lyons and co-workers (26) investigated 17 subjects with category 2 and 3 simple coal workers' pneumoconiosis, divided into those with p and m lesions on the chest radiograph. They used the single-breath technique and found that 10 of the 16 with pinpoint lesions had reduced D_L and pulmonary capillary blood volume, whereas the 11 subjects with micronodular opacities all showed normal values. There were, however, more smokers in the group with pinpoint lesions, and when this factor was corrected for the difference between the groups, though still present, was only significant at the 7% level.

Twenty-one subjects studied in the Appalachian Laboratory for Occupational Respiratory Diseases were selected on the basis that they were working coal miners, did not smoke, and had no obstructive airway disease. All had category 2 or 3 simple pneumoconiosis. The single-breath D_L was calculated, using the body plethysmograph rather than helium dilution for determination of residual volume. This results in values for D_L rather higher than in other reported series. The prediction formula for D_L by this technique in our laboratory is $D_L = 1.48 \times$ height (in.) $- 64.03$. In Table VI the mean values obtained in this series are summarized. All subjects studied had a normal D_L, but D_L/TLC differed significantly between the two groups, being lower in those with the pinpoint type of lesion ($t = 1.55$, $p < 0.05$).

TABLE VI

SINGLE-BREATH DIFFUSING CAPACITY IN UNOBSTRUCTED SUBJECTS WITH SIMPLE CWP

Category	Number of subjects		Age (years)	Height (cms)	Surface area (m²)	TLC (liters)	D_L (ml/min/mm Hg)		D_L/TLC	$\dfrac{D_L \text{ pred}}{D_L \text{ obs}}$ (%)
							Pred	Obsd		
p	6	Mean	57	176	1.96	6.58	40	38	5.7	93
		S.D.	(7)	(6.3)	(0.12)	(0.69)	(5.5)	(6.2)	(0.6)	(8.6)
m	15	Mean	56	175	1.97	6.43	41	41	6.4	101
		S.D.	(5)	(3.8)	(0.15)	(1.05)	(3.6)	(6.0)	(0.7)	(11.8)

Sixteen coal workers with complicated stages-B and -C pneumoconiosis were also studied in this laboratory, using the steady-state method. There were eight subjects in each group, and there was no significant difference between the groups in terms of age or height. Those with stage B pneumoconiosis had slightly more airway obstruction. The mean D_L, expressed as a percentage of predicted normal, was 47.1% in those with category B and 47.2% in those with stage C. In the six patients with only minor or no obstruction ($FEV_1/FVC > 60\%$) the mean D_L was 48%. The results in this series are given in Table VII.

TABLE VII
STEADY-STATE DIFFUSING CAPACITY IN SUBJECTS WITH COMPLICATED CWP

Stage	Number of subjects		Age (years)	Height (cm)	$\dfrac{FEV_1}{FVC}$ %	D_L (ml/min/mm Hg) Pred	Obsd	D_L % Pred
B	8	Mean	65	171	48	25	12	47
		S.D.	(8)	(6)	(17)	(7)	(5)	(10)
C	8	Mean	60	171	63	23	11	47
		S.D.	(9)	(5)	(15)	(5)	(6)	(21)

In most of these investigations there has not been a clear definition of the type of problem being studied, and this may partly explain the discrepancies between the results of different authors. True silicosis may undoubtedly cause obliteration of the pulmonary capillary bed and alveolar distortion with resultant lowering of D_L, but silicosis occurs relatively uncommonly in coal workers in the United States. Also, bronchitis and emphysema may cause a reduction in D_L, and therefore if the effects of coal workers' pneumoconiosis are being studied, such patients should be excluded. Cigarette smokers may have a relatively high back pressure of carbon monoxide, and unless this is measured it may lead to incorrect results using the single-breath technique. The single-breath technique is also dependent on a measurement of residual volume, and if this is high, as has been described in coal workers, an artificially high D_L may result. The steady-state method may also be misleading if the subject hyperventilates, though expressing the results as D_L divided by tidal volume may overcome this. This method is also more satisfactory for exercise studies.

In summary, D_L is reduced relatively infrequently in subjects with simple coal workers' pneumoconiosis. It seems likely that there is a difference between subjects with p and m types of simple pneumoconiosis, those with p lesions having lower values of D_L, and this may be related to some diminution of the pulmonary capillary bed. Complicating bronchitis and emphysema or the presence of silicosis rather than coal workers' pneumoconiosis may also cause a lower D_L. In complicated pneumoconiosis, by contrast, the D_L is frequently much lower than the predicted normal.

Gas Exchange

Studies of gas exchange among United States coal workers have been limited for the most part to symptomatic subjects. Motley and co-workers (3) reported the results of their studies of respiratory gas exchange in 100 symptomatic anthracite-coal miners. They classified the subjects into groups having no, slight, moderate, advanced, and far-advanced emphysema on the basis of the RV/TLC ratio. Mean resting arterial carbon dioxide tension ($P_a CO_2$) and content were elevated in the subjects with abnormally increased RV/TLC; however, the arterial pH was also elevated, indicating that the subjects were acclimated to the higher $P_a CO_2$ levels and in some instances were hyperventilating at the time of the study. The mean resting arterial oxygen tension ($P_a O_2$) was subnormal in all groups with a slightly greater decrease in the patients with advanced and far-advanced emphysema. The arterial blood-oxygen saturation was also subnormal, but only in the advanced and far-advanced categories was there a further decrease with increasing RV/TLC. The resting oxygen gradient ($A–a)O_2$ was abnormally increased in all subjects, and no linear association between increasing gradient and RV/TLC abnormality was evident. During exercise there was a progressive increase in CO_2 content and a decrease in O_2 saturation that correlated well with increasing RV/TLC. Studies with low- and high-oxygen inspired gas mixtures indicated that the hypoxemia and increased oxygen gradient were the result of unequal ventilation and perfusion rather than abnormalities of diffusion.

Measurements of oxygen consumption, carbon dioxide production, and minute ventilation at rest were approximately the same for all groups of symptomatic anthracite miners. The average minute ventilation during exercise in the subjects with the largest RV/TLC ratios tended to be slightly lower than for subjects with normal or slightly increased RV/TLC ratios. This lack of ability to increase ventilation with exercise in the subjects with increased RV/TLC ratios no doubt contributed to their worsening gas exchange.

Motley (27) also studied ventilation and respiratory gas exchange in 56 symptomatic bituminous-coal miners. These subjects were also grouped according to RV/TLC ratio into those with no, slight, moderate, advanced, and far-advanced emphysema. The findings observed in these subjects were similar to those observed in anthracite miners. Subjects with increased RV/TLC ratios in general showed increased arterial CO_2 content and pH at rest with a decreased O_2 tension and saturation in the more severely abnormal groups. The mean resting $(A-a)O_2$ gradient also tended to increase with increasing abnormality of the RV/TLC ratio. During exercise these abnormalities were accentuated and in general correlated quite well with increasing abnormality of the RV/TLC ratio. As was the case with anthracite miners, the abnormalities of gas exchange were largely the result of unequal ventilation and perfusion rather than impairment of diffusion. The subjects with the largest RV/TLC ratios demonstrated lower minute ventilation during exercise than those with less severe impairment of RV/TLC ratio. Minute ventilation, oxygen uptake, and carbon dioxide production both at rest and with exercise did not differ among the various groups.

Twenty-five symptomatic, nonworking miners from Pennsylvania, West Virginia, and Ohio were studied by Ferris and Frank (12). These miners ranged in age from 47 to 71 years. Six subjects with complicated pneumoconiosis had the most striking abnormalities in lung volumes and airflow resistance. The eight patients with category 2 and 3 simple pneumoconiosis showed the most abnormal blood gases, but a number also had bullous changes which may have contributed to this. When the patients were grouped according to mild, moderate, and severe impairment based upon the airflow resistance values, there was a general tendency for abnormalities in arterial oxygen tension, saturation and $(A-a)O_2$ gradient to correlate with increasing airflow resistance.

Rasmussen and co-workers (8) studied the ventilatory function, respiratory gas exchange, and work capacity of 192 symptomatic bituminous-coal miners from southern West Virginia. Mean values for lung volumes, ventilatory capacity, and intrapulmonary mixing of inspired air showed little correlation with radiographic category when the subjects were grouped without regard to the presence or absence of airflow obstruction. There was, however, a tendency for arterial oxygen tension to decrease and the $(A-a)O_2$ gradient to increase with increasing category of pneumoconiosis in the group as a whole.

When the subjects were grouped into those with "normal" and those with "abnormal" ventilatory capacity on the basis of an FEV_1/FVC ratio of greater or less than 75%, several differences became apparent. The mean value for arterial oxygen tension was lower and the mean values for $(A-a)O_2$ gradient and physiological dead space/tidal volume (V_D/V_T) ratio were higher in those with abnormal ventilatory capacity. When the subjects with abnormal ventilatory capacity were grouped according to radiographic category, there were no significant differences in these same parameters between the groups. Among the subjects with normal ventilatory capacity, there were, however, fairly large differences in arterial oxygen tension and $(A–a)O_2$ gradients between the radiographic categories with a general trend towards increasing abnormality with increasing radiographic evidence of pneumoconiosis. Hyperventilation during exercise was present in all groups with little difference between radiographic categories and tended to be higher in those with normal ventilatory capacity than in those with impaired ventilatory capacity.

Henschel (9) studied the work capacity and some aspects of gas exchange in five groups of subjects as part of a prevalence survey for pneumoconiosis. There were 1666 working miners who completed the entire series of graded exercise. In two West Virginia communities, Richwood and Mullens, smaller groups of working miners were compared with groups of nonminers. The indices selected by which to compare groups were pulse rate, oxygen consumption, and minute ventilation. Henschel concluded that working miners were not significantly different from nonminers in their response to graded exercise. This conclusion is at variance with that of Enterline (28), who found a significantly lower ventilatory capacity among working miners in Mullens as compared to age-matched nonminers from the same community. One reason for this disparity of findings may be that Enterline included only matched pairs in his study, while Henschel included additional volunteers who were not selected in the random sample (28a).

Fifty-one symptomatic coal miners who demonstrated no significant obstruction as determined by an FEV_1/FVC ratio of greater than 70% underwent studies of gas exchange at the Appalachian Laboratory for Occupational Respiratory Diseases. Their chest radiographs were classified as showing complicated pneumoconiosis stage A in three subjects, and category 0, 1, 2, or 3 simple pneumoconiosis in the remainder. The results are shown in Table VIII. Subjects with categories 0 and 1 demonstrated mean arterial oxygen tensions that were slightly reduced at rest but which returned to normal on exercise. The mean arterial oxygen tension during exercise was normal for all the groups, although occasional subjects did demonstrate decreases. The mean value for alveolar–arterial oxygen gradient was abnormally elevated in the subjects with category 0, but decreased into the normal range with exercise. The mean value for physiological dead-space/tidal-volume ratio (V_D/V_T) was abnormally high at rest in all groups but returned to normal on exercise except in the group with category 3 and in those with complicated pneumoconiosis. Minute ventilation was high at rest in all groups, but only in the subjects with category 3 and complicated pneumoconiosis was there hyperventilation during exercise. These results indicate that abnormalities of dis-

TABLE VIII

GAS EXCHANGE IN SUBJECTS WITH SIMPLE CWP

Radiographic category	Number of patients		Age	(A–a) O$_2$ (mm Hg)		P$_a$O$_2$ (mm Hg)		V$_D$/V$_T$		Minute ventilation (L/min/m^2)		Oxygen uptake (L/min/m^2)	
				Rest	Exer.	Rest	Exer.	Rest	Exer.	Rest	Exer.	Rest	Exer.
0	12	Mean	53	32	25	76	81	0.43	0.35	6.69	19.73	0.158	0.587
		S.D.	(12.2)	(12.8)	(7.8)	(11.1)	(6.5)	(0.10)	(0.15)	(1.40)	(4.76)	(0.027)	(0.168)
1	23	Mean	59	24	24	77	80	0.45	0.35	6.18	19.13	0.156	0.540
		S.D.	(4.9)	(12.3)	(11.9)	(9.5)	(9.1)	(0.12)	(0.09)	(1.54)	(8.21)	(0.034)	(0.171)
2	11	Mean	55	24	30	81	82	0.49	0.37	6.86	20.93	0.152	0.555
		S.D.	(7.4)	(12.4)	(19.4)	(8.4)	(8.5)	(0.08)	(0.11)	(2.41)	(7.09)	(0.040)	(0.327)
3 and A	5	Mean	55	27	30	82	81	0.40	0.40	5.87	27.37	0.134	0.629
		S.D.	(9.5)	(8.6)	(18.1)	(6.1)	(16.7)	(0.06)	(0.14)	(1.61)	(11.60)	(0.018)	(0.152)

tribution and gas exchange may occur in the absence of gross airway obstruction in symptomatic coal miners whose chest radiographs demonstrate no evidence of pneumoconiosis. This may be a consequence of focal emphysema or of airflow obstruction in small airways that is not detected by the conventional ventilatory tests.

Fourteen symptomatic coal miners with complicated pneumoconiosis classified as stage B or C underwent studies of respiratory gas exchange at the Appalachian Laboratory for Occupational Respiratory Diseases. All were studied at rest as well as during exercise. The results of these studies are shown in Table IX. As generally occurs in symptomatic miners with advanced complicated pneumoconiosis, our subjects demonstrated mean FEV_1/FVC ratios that were abnormally low. Their $(A-a)O_2$ gradients rose abnormally with exercise, while their arterial oxygen tensions during exercise tended to decrease rather than increase or remain unchanged, as was the case with the miners with simple pneumoconiosis and no major airflow obstruction. The mean values for V_D/V_T ratio were abnormally elevated at rest in the miners with categories B and C pneumoconiosis, and on exercise this ratio did not return to normal, as it did in most of the miners with simple pneumoconiosis.

In summary, symptomatic miners with normal ventilatory capacity tend to have abnormalities of respiratory gas exchange that are the result of abnormal ventilation–perfusion relationships. While there is a general tendency for the gas exchange abnormalities to increase with increasing category of pneumoconiosis, the association is not always present. These abnormalities tend to be more severe in subjects with a decreased ventilatory capacity. Measurements of gas exchange in working asymptomatic miners have been made relatively infrequently.

Hemodynamics

Pathologic studies have in general shown cor pulmonale to be an infrequent sequel to simple coal workers' pneumoconiosis in the absence of chronic bronchitis or other complicating respiratory diseases (29–31). Studies of hemodynamics carried out on coal workers have mostly supported these conclusions. Bollinelli *et al.* (32) documented pulmonary hypertension in a selected group of 15 subjects with complicated "silicosis," contrasting the results with those in 16 simple "silicotics," five of whom had a raised pulmonary artery pressure on exercise. These authors considered the high pressure to be related to both anatomic restriction of the pulmonary bed and to arterial desaturation. Stoeckle and his colleagues (33) reported in outline the results of cardiac catheterization in 17 disabled Appalachian miners, finding no evidence of right ven-

TABLE IX

Gas Exchange in Subjects with Complicated CWP

Radiographic category	Number of subjects		Age	$(A-a)O_2$ (mm Hg)		$P_a O_2$ (mm Hg)		V_D/V_T		Minute ventilation (L/min/m²)		Oxygen uptake (L/min/m²)		$\dfrac{FEV_1}{FVC} \times 100$
				Rest	Exer.	Rest	Exer.	Rest	Exer.	Rest	Exer.	Rest	Exer.	
B	7	Mean	63	29	31	74	71	0.51	0.40	5.50	16.20	0.148	0.476	57
		S.D.	(8.8)	(14.4)	(12.5)	(6.3)	(14.2)	(0.08)	(0.14)	(1.23)	(5.68)	(0.029)	(0.139)	(19.5)
C	7	Mean	53	25	35	76	64	0.52	0.43	6.42	17.05	0.150	0.476	65
		S.D.	(6.1)	(7.4)	(11.6)	(11.1)	(7.6)	(0.10)	(0.08)	(1.13)	(8.08)	(0.047)	(0.224)	(11.5)

tricular failure, although eight had slightly raised pulmonary vascular resistances and 12 showed some elevation of pulmonary artery pressure after 2 minutes of exercise.

Kremer and co-workers (34, 35) showed that pulmonary artery pressure in coal workers was related to the degree of airway obstruction and that pulmonary artery pressure in miners with obstructive airway disease was no higher than in similarly obstructed nonmining bronchitics. They demonstrated a statistical increase in the pulmonary artery pressures of a group of miners with categories 2m and 3m pneumoconiosis as compared to a similar group of normal subjects and miners with category 1 pneumoconiosis. None of their unobstructed subjects with simple pneumoconiosis had a raised pulmonary artery pressure. They also concluded that both restriction of the vascular bed and hypoxemia played a part in production of the cardiac disorder. Podlesch and co-workers (23) catheterized 16 "silicotic" subjects and found the pulmonary artery pressure to be raised in those with obstructive bronchitis. A moderate increase in pressure on exercise was noted in all subjects, only occasionally accompanied by any fall in arterial oxygen tension.

Rasmussen and co-workers (8) suggested on the basis of tests of gas exchange that pulmonary hypertension might be more frequent in American coal workers, and they demonstrated high systolic pulmonary artery pressure in several subjects. Mean pressures and pulmonary vascular resistances were not recorded, however, so unequivocal evidence of cor pulmonale was not obtained. Stanescu (36) raised other objections to certain aspects of this study. Cotes (37) reported a significantly higher mean pulmonary artery pressure in five subjects with coal workers' pneumoconiosis and bronchitis than in five similar subjects without bronchitis. Navratil (38) found pulmonary hypertension in one of 24 subjects with simple or complicated category A pneumoconiosis and in five of 23 miners with complicated category B or C pneumoconiosis. He also demonstrated a correlation between forced expiratory volume in 1 second and mean pulmonary artery pressure, but he failed to differentiate between those of his patients with coal workers' pneumoconiosis and those with silicosis.

Lapp et al. (39) studied 47 symptomatic Appalachian coal workers. The details of mean pulmonary artery pressures and arterial oxygen tensions at rest and on exercise are illustrated in Figs. 3 and 4. Seven of 24 subjects with airway obstruction had pulmonary hypertension that could be accounted for either by the airway disease or by complicated pneumoconiosis. Of the 23 men without airway obstruction, many of whom had marked abnormalities of gas exchange, only one had pulmonary hypertension at rest and three others had an abnormal elevation on exercise.

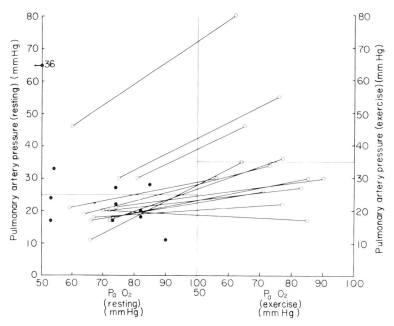

FIG. 3. Data for coal miners with obstructive airway disease. (Left panel) This shows the mean pulmonary artery pressure versus resting arterial oxygen tension in coal miners with obstructive airway disease. (Right panel) This shows the mean pulmonary artery pressure versus the arterial oxygen tension during exercise. The horizontal lines at 25 mm Hg in the left panel and 35 mm Hg in the right panel are the upper limits that we accepted as normal for pulmonary artery pressure under these conditions. The open circles represent subjects studied at rest and on exercise. The closed circles represent subjects studied only at rest. [*From* Pulmonary hemodynamics in coal workers' pneumoconiosis *in* "Inhaled Particles and Vapors" (H. Walton, ed.), Vol. III. Unwin Brothers Limited, Old Woking, Surrey, England, to be published 1971.]

These four all had the pinpoint (p) type of radiographic lesion, and two of them had been exposed to silica in their work. In addition, one other subject with airway obstruction had a raised pulmonary artery pressure in spite of only mild obstruction, and he likewise had the p type of opacity present ($2p$). In this study, there was a significant negative correlation between mean pulmonary artery pressure at rest and forced expiratory volume in 1 second expressed as a percentage of forced vital capacity.

Seaton and co-workers (40) used the technique of lung scanning with macroaggregates of albumin to investigate the pulmonary microcirculation in coal workers. They found areas of absent perfusion related to areas of conglomeration and bullae in all of 16 subjects with complicated pneumoconiosis, but only minor abnormalities in two out of 21 subjects with simple pneumoconiosis.

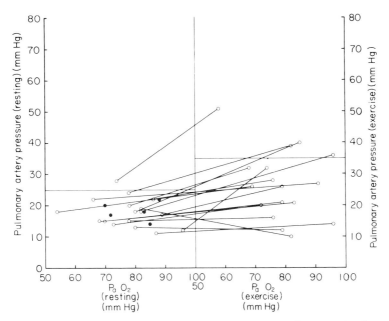

FIG. 4. Data for coal miners without obstructive airway disease. The format is the same as Fig. 3 with resting mean pulmonary artery pressure versus arterial oxygen tension in the left panel and exercise mean pulmonary artery pressure versus arterial oxygen tension in the right panel. The horizontal lines at 25 mm Hg in the left panel and 35 mm Hg in the right panel are the upper limits we accepted as normal for pulmonary artery pressure under these conditions. The open circles represent subjects studied at rest and on exercise. The closed circles represent subjects studied at rest only. [*From* Pulmonary hemodynamics in coal workers' pneumoconiosis *in* "Inhaled Particles and Vapors" (H. Walton, ed.), Vol. III. Unwin Brothers Limited, Old Woking, Surrey, England, to be published 1971.]

Coal workers, therefore, appear liable to develop cor pulmonale if their pneumoconiosis is of the complicated type or if they have silicosis or chronic bronchitis. Simple pneumoconiosis per se appears to be associated with pulmonary hypertension only rarely, even though definite abnormalities of gas exchange may be present. However, it is possible that those subjects with pinpoint lesions on the chest radiograph may be more liable to develop pulmonary hypertension. This, considered with the finding mentioned in a previous section—a lowered D_L in such subjects—suggests that this lesion may occasionally cause restriction of the pulmonary vascular bed.

Conclusions

The coal miner with simple pneumoconiosis is likely to have a slight reduction in ventilatory capacity. It becomes more marked if he smokes or if he is over 50 years of age. His pulmonary mechanics and diffusing capacity are likely to be normal unless he has bronchitis and emphysema. He may have a slight increase in (A–a) oxygen gradient and a decrease in arterial oxygen tension at rest, but these will be corrected by exercise. In the absence of chronic bronchitis or other concomitant pulmonary disease, he is most unlikely to have pulmonary hypertension.

The miner with stage B or C complicated pneumoconiosis, on the other hand, will generally have a marked reduction in ventilatory capacity, a low diffusing capacity, and abnormalities of gas exchange. He is liable to develop pulmonary hypertension, even in the absence of severe airway obstruction. His pulmonary mechanics may indicate either increased or decreased compliance, depending on the relative proportions of emphysema and fibrosis.

Certain aspects of pulmonary function in coal workers' pneumoconiosis remain unclear in the light of present knowledge. The precise relationship of airway obstruction to pneumoconiosis is ill defined. In particular, the effect of smoking and the inhalation of toxic vapors on the deposition of dust and on the development of pneumoconiosis deserves further study. The causes of the abnormalities of gas exchange so frequently found are unclear and might be elucidated by studies of regional ventilation and perfusion with radioactive gases. It may be that the lesion in coal workers' pneumoconiosis causes a functional disturbance of the small peripheral airways and that this is responsible for alteration of distribution and, hence, the blood gas abnormalities. Studies of the effect on compliance of increasing respiratory rates might be of use to test this hypothesis. Finally, there appears to be a physiological difference between different types of radiographic lesion. Further investigation of this, and in particular of its pathologic basis, may prove worthwhile.

ACKNOWLEDGMENTS

The authors wish to acknowledge the assistance of Mr. Edward J. Baier, Director, Division of Occupational Health, Pennsylvania Department of Occupational Health, and Dr. James Walker of the West Virginia State Silicosis Board in obtaining subjects with complicated pneumoconiosis.

REFERENCES

1. International Labour Office (1959). "International Classification of Radiographs of Pneumoconiosis." Occup. Saf. Health, Geneva, Switzerland.
2. Motley, H. L., Lang, L. P., and Gordon, B. (1949). Amer. Rev. Tuberc. 59, 270.
3. Motley, H. L., Lang, L. P., and Gordon, B. (1950). Amer. Rev. Tuberc. 61, 201.
4. Pemberton, J. (1956). Arch. Ind. Health 13, 529.
5. Anderson, W. H., Gilbert, L. H., and Dossett, B. E. (1960). Arch. Environ. Health 1, 540.

6. Hyatt, R. E., Kistin, A. D., and Mahan, T. K. (1964). *Amer. Rev. Resp. Dis.* **89**, 387.
7. Higgins, I. T. T., *et al.* (1968). *Brit. J. Ind. Med.* **25**, 165.
8. Rasmussen, D. L., *et al.* (1968). *Amer. Rev. Resp. Dis.* **98**, 658.
9. Henschel, A. (1969). "Ventilatory Function and Work Capacity in Appalachian Bituminous Coal Miners and Miners and Non-Miners in Two West Virginia Communities, *in* Pneumoconiosis in Appalachian Bituminous Coal Miners." Govt. Print. Off., Washington, D. C.
10. Morgan, W. K. C., *et al.* (1971). *Thorax* (in press).
11. Leathart, G. L. (1959). *Brit. J. Ind. Med.* **16**, 153.
12. Ferris, B. G., and Frank, N. R. (1962). *J. Occup. Med.* **4**, 274.
13. Schleuter, D. P., Immekus, J., and Stead, W. W. (1967). *Amer. Rev. Resp. Dis.* **96**, 656.
14. Woolcock, A. J., Vincent, N. J., and Macklem, P. T. (1969). *J. Clin. Invest.* **48**, 1097.
15. Macklem, P. T., and Mead, J. (1967). *J. Appl. Physiol.* **22**, 395.
16. Gilson, J. C., and Hugh-Jones, P. (1955). *Med. Res. Counc. Gt. Brit. Spec. Rep. Ser.* 290.
17. Gaensler, E. A., Hoffman, L., and Elliott, M. F. (1960). *Poumon Coeur* **16**, 1137.
18. Sartorelli, E., *et al.* (1963). *Med. Lav.* **54**, 191.
19. Billiet, L., *et al.* (1964). *Acta Tuberc. Pneumol. Belg.* **55**, 255.
20. Englert, M., and DeCoster, A. (1965). *J. Fr. Med. Chir. Thorac.* **19**, 159.
21. Vanroux, R., and Gregoire, M. (1965). *Lille Med.* **10**, 129.
22. Lavenne, F., Meersseman, F., and Brasseur, L. (1964). *Rev. Inst. Hyg. Mines* **20**, 33.
23. Podlesch, I., Stevanovic, M., and Ulmer, W. T. (1966). *Med. Thorac.* **23**, 283.
24. Nicaise, R., Vereerstraeten, J., and DeClercq, F. (1967). *Proc. Roy. Ned. Tuberc. Ass.* **10**, 70.
25. Ogilvie, C., Brown, K., and Kearns, W. E. (1967). *Brit. Med. J.* **3**, 10.
26. Lyons, J. P., *et al.* (1967). *Brit. Med. J.* **4**, 772.
27. Motley, H. L. (1950). *W. Va. Med. J.* **46**, 8.
28. Enterline, P. E. (1969). "Prevalence of Respiratory Symptoms in Two Appalachian Communities, *in* Pneumoconiosis in Appalachian Bituminous Coal Miners." Govt. Print. Off., Washington, D. C.
28a. Enterline, P. E. Personal communication.
29. Thomas, A. J. (1948). *Brit. Heart J.* **10**, 282.
30. Thomas, A. J. (1951). *Brit. Heart J.* **13**, 1.
31. Wells, A. L. (1954). *J. Pathol. Bacteriol.* **68**, 573.
32. Bollinelli, R., Le Tallec, Y., and Bollinelli, M. (1957). *J. Fr. Med. Chir. Thorac.* **11**, 594.
33. Stoeckle, J. D., *et al.* (1962). *J. Chronic Dis.* **15**, 887.
34. Kremer, R., and Lavenne, F. (1966). *Poumon Coeur* **22**, 767.
35. Kremer, R., *et al.* (1967). *Rev. Inst. Hyg. Mines* **22**, 3.
36. Stanescu, D. (1969). *Amer. Rev. Resp. Dis.* **100**, 106.
37. Cotes, J. E. (1968). *Bull. Physio. Pathol. Resp.* **4**, 207.
38. Navratil, M., Widimski, J., and Kasalicky, J. (1968). *Bull. Physio. Pathol. Resp.* **4**, 349.
39. Lapp, N. L., *et al.* (1971). "Pulmonary Hemodynamics in Coal Workers' Pneumoconiosis." *Amer. Rev. Resp. Dis.* (in press).
40. Seaton, A., Lapp, N. L., and Chang, C. H. (1971). "Lung Perfusion Scanning in Coal Workers' Pneumoconiosis." *Amer. Rev. Resp. Dis.* **103**, 338.

9

Complications

R. W. Penman

Progressive Massive Fibrosis (PMF)

This complication is liable to occur in more advanced cases of pneumoconiosis due to coal dust, silica, kaolin, hematite, or graphite. The condition is characterized by widespread consolidation composed of large amounts of dust enmeshed in connective tissue. The chest radiograph shows rounded masses, often several centimeters in diameter, in one or both upper lobes. Central cavitation is frequently seen within these masses of fibrous tissue.

Studies of random samples of coal miners in the United States (U. S. Public Health Service, unpublished data) have shown the prevalence of PMF to be approximately one-third of all cases of CWP. However, there is considerable geographic variation, possibly due to variations in mining conditions and in the age and work experience of the mining populations in different areas (1–4). The rate at which simple pneumoconiosis gives rise to PMF and the rate of progression of PMF from its early to its later stages have not been measured in the United States. British experience suggests that about 1% of men with simple CWP develop PMF each year and that of those with PMF, about 5% show some progression in severity. It is well established that PMF is much more likely to develop in those with categories 2 or 3 simple pneumoconiosis than in those with category 1 and that PMF may develop in men with advanced simple pneumoconiosis in the absence of further dust exposure. Thus, it has been suggested many times that some factor other than the mere physical presence of dust in the lungs is important in the development of PMF. In the past, tuberculous infection was thought to be the most important factor, but the general decline in incidence of tuberculosis has not been accompanied by a similar decline in PMF. Furthermore, a trial of antituberculous chemotherapy as a prophylactic measure in coal miners has failed to influence the development of PMF (5), and other studies have shown no difference in the tuberculin reaction to 5 TU between miners and ex-miners with PMF and men with simple or no pneumoconiosis (6).

Other workers have suggested that the development of PMF bears some relationship to the silica content of the lungs. As evidence for this theory it is pointed out that PMF occurs more frequently, and with greater severity, in cases of classical silicosis than in coal workers' pneumoconiosis. However, chemical studies of the lungs of coal miners with PMF have shown that only 2–3% of the usual 40–50 g of dust is quartz (7), and Nagelschmidt has found (8) that although the dust content of PMF lesions is about twice as high as in the rest of the lung, the quartz content is not significantly different.

Various other theories have been advanced to explain the etiology of PMF. At present it is widely held that PMF results from the interaction of dust and host factors including an immune reaction. In the case of classical silicosis it has been shown (9) that the death of silica laden macrophages results in the liberation of phospholipids which are fibrogenic. Other factors, including products from tubercle or other bacilli, may act in the manner of a "Freund's Adjuvant" to boost the immunity response (10).

The clinical features of progressive massive fibrosis are similar to those seen with fibrosis due to other types of lung disease (tuberculosis, collagen disorders, etc.). Thus, the earliest symptom is dyspnea on exertion which becomes more severe as the lesion progresses. In many cases, a coexisting chronic bronchitis and/or emphysema aggravates the disability. With the onset of PMF the disorders of pulmonary gas exchange which occur in simple pneumoconiosis are increased, and cyanosis and clubbing of the extremities may appear. The victim exhibits tachypnea, and chest movement is seen to be restricted, leading to inadequate alveolar ventilation with a consequent increase in arterial carbon dioxide tension, at first on exercise and later at rest. At this stage, evidence of cor pulmonale may be found on clinical examination or on the electrocardiogram, and this may be accompanied by frank congestive cardiac failure. The lesions of PMF are permanent, and there is no evidence that the frequently relentless progression through these clinical stages can be influenced by any treatment.

Caplan's Syndrome

In 1953 Caplan (11) drew attention to the presence of nodular densities in the lungs of Welsh coal miners with rheumatoid arthritis. Since then, there have been numerous reports in the European and American literature of this association. The nodules usually measure 5–15 mm in diameter, and they may develop rapidly in the presence of little or no radiographic evidence of pneumoconiosis (12). The nodules may conglomerate into larger masses measuring 5 cm or more in diameter. Ultimately, cavitation may occur in these larger lesions. Gough (13) tells of the problem of identifying the origin of these nodules prior to Caplan's observation of their association with rheumatoid arthritis; he observes that in the United States these lesions were commonly attributed to histoplasmosis infection, although *Histoplasma capsulatum* could not be demonstrated in the lesions.

The morphology of these nodules is characteristic. There are concentric rings of light and dark material, the lighter area being zones of active inflammation and necrosis, the darker areas being composed largely of coal dust. The severity of the lung changes is not proportional to the severity of the arthritis. Some severe cases of arthritis show no pulmonary lesions, and some cases with severe lung changes occur with only slight arthritis. In several cases these nodules have been shown to disappear on serial chest X rays, but more commonly they become incorporated in large areas of fibrosis which are indistinguishable from PMF.

The etiology of these characteristic nodules in the lungs of coal workers with rheumatoid arthritis is presumably that of an immune reaction involving a rheumatoid factor or factors and coal dust. The role of the dust in the reaction appears to be nonspecific since similar lesions have been observed in the lungs of workers exposed to dust in potteries and from sandblasting and in brass and iron foundries and other industries. Further research in the area of etiology of Caplan's syndrome may have important implications for the etiology of PMF and even simple pneumoconiosis in which potent "host factors" have long been suspected.

Progressive Systemic Sclerosis (Scleroderma)

In 1914, Bramwell (14) reported five cases of scleroderma occurring in stonemasons and one in a coal miner. He speculated on the possible association between these occupations and scleroderma. In 1959, Erasmus reported a high incidence of scleroderma in South Africa goldminers (15). In these cases the disease was characterized by an acute onset of pulmonary manifestations leading to severe disability. There was also a frequent association with myocardial infarction.

In this country, Rodman (16) has drawn attention to a similar increased incidence of scleroderma among coal miners and others with siliceous dust exposure. The great majority of these cases exhibited no signs of pneumoconiosis. Unlike Erasmus, Rodman found no unusual features in the presentation or course of the disease.

The nature of the relationship between coal workers' pneumoconiosis or silicosis and scleroderma remains obscure. Vigliani and Pernis (17) have postulated "a reciprocal potentiation" between these conditions, and this supports the impression of Erasmus (15) that "the degree of disability in most cases was too severe for a purely additive effect."

Cor Pulmonale

The term cor pulmonale is conventionally applied when there is evidence of right ventricular enlargement resulting from a disorder of the lungs. The mechanism of the right ventricular enlargement is related to the abnormal load which pulmonary hypertension imposes on the right ventricle. This load is aggravated by the occasional occurrence of a high cardiac output. Signs of right ventricular enlargement may be detected on clinical examination or on electrocardiography. The latter has been shown to be a reasonably accurate method of predicting the thickness of the right ventricular wall at autopsy. More severe degrees of right ventricular hypertrophy commonly progress to failure of the right heart with clinical signs of congestive cardiac failure.

By far the most frequent cause of cor pulmonale in coal miners, as in the general population, is that group of diseases which lead to inefficiency of pulmonary gas exchange, i.e., chronic bronchitis, emphysema, asthma, and pulmonary fibrosis. The pulmonary hypertension which often occurs in these conditions appears to be largely a consequence of hypoxia and carbon dioxide retention. Anatomical restriction of the pulmonary vascular bed plays a comparatively minor part, along with an increased cardiac output in a few cases. Thus, numerous studies have shown that the cardiac output must be increased threefold above the resting value before pulmonary artery pressures increase and that almost two-thirds of the lungs must be removed before there is any appreciable pulmonary hypertension at rest. On the other hand, pulmonary artery pressure is significantly increased, due to vasoconstriction, whenever the arterial oxygen saturation falls below 80%, and this effect is potentiated by an increase in arterial carbon dioxide tension (18).

Aside from the well-known association of cor pulmonale with the chronic lung diseases which occur in both miners and nonminers, there has been no satisfactory study of the association of cor pulmonale and simple coal workers' pneumoconiosis. Lavenne (19) noted that cor pulmonale occurred in coal miners independently of the presence or absence of pneumoconiosis. He stressed the need for studies to assess whether or not pulmonary hypertension occurred with lesser degrees of chronic airway obstruction in miners with chronic bronchitis or emphysema and associated pneumoconiosis. Rasmussen and co-workers (20) have suggested that there may be an abnormal response of pulmonary artery pressure and of the "dead space" ventilation of the lungs in response to exercise on the part of miners with or without radiological evidence of simple pneumoconiosis. If this suggestion is confirmed with suitable control observations, it would point to a considerable restriction of the pulmonary vascular bed in coal miners.

In contrast to the present uncertainty regarding the association of simple pneumoconiosis and cor pulmonale, it is generally agreed that the lesions of PMF are frequently associated with right ventricular enlargement and a high mortality from frank congestive cardiac failure. Presumably this association reflects the severe derangements of pulmonary gas exchange in PMF together with the widespread obliteration of the pulmonary capillary bed due to masses of fibrous tissue. In many of these cases there is also a concomitant chronic bronchitis and emphysema which may play a larger part in the development of cor pulmonale.

Emphysema

"Emphysema" is a frequent clinical diagnosis. In this country, until very recently, the term was applied to any patient with chronic obstructive lung disease. Many of these cases would now be given a diagnosis of chronic bronchitis. Autopsy studies have shown that there may be no evidence of anatomic emphysema in spite of severe airway obstruction during life. On the other hand, it is now also apparent that severe emphysema may be present in many persons who have no significant airway obstruction (21–24). This confusion of clinical and pathological terms has been a major obstacle to progress in the differentiation of the chronic obstructive lung diseases, and it has complicated the study of the relationships between pneumoconiosis and chronic lung disease. There is now general agreement that pulmonary emphysema should be defined in anatomical terms as a condition of the lungs characterized by increase beyond the normal in the size of air spaces distal to the terminal bronchiole. Opinions differ whether the term should be restricted to cases where the enlargement of air spaces is due to destruction of alveolar walls (25, 26) or should include cases with mere dilatation without destruction of the alveoli (27).

There is reason to believe that three types of emphysema are of special significance in a study of CWP. These are focal, centrilobular, and panlobular emphysema. The term *focal dust emphysema* describes an enlargement of air spaces in and around deposits of dust (28, 29). Dilatation of the respiratory bronchioles occurs in the vicinity of the simple coal nodule. Subsequent shrinkage of the dust foci leads to enlargement of the peribronchiolar air spaces which is termed focal emphysema.

Centrilobular emphysema occurs both in miners and nonminers. As with focal dust emphysema, it affects the center of the respiratory lobules. It is a consequence of bronchiolitis (30), and the evidence of bronchiolar inflammation may be seen histologically. If widespread, this form of emphysema gives rise to severe functional disturbances of gas exchange, and it is responsible for much of the progression of chronic nonspecific lung disease into the stage of cor pulmonale. At the present time, it is uncertain what part dust exposure may play in the development of centrilobular emphysema in coal miners' lungs. It appears unlikely that dust retention, per se, without accompanying infection of the terminal airways, could lead to this condition. (*Editor's note:* Cf. Chap. 5.)

Panlobular emphysema is the type which is characterized by dilation and destruction of the entire acinus distal to the respiratory bronchiole. Inflammation and distortion of the bronchioles is inconspicuous in panlobular emphysema as compared with the findings in centrilobular emphysema. It is likely that this contrast reflects an entirely different pathological process, although both conditions frequently coexist, suggesting the possibility of a common factor. Unlike focal and centrilobular emphysema, this type is readily diagnosed during life from radiographic changes (31). Panlobular emphysema is such a common condition in the population at large that it is difficult to determine whether it bears any significant relationship to CWP. Individual cases of CWP which have been followed for a number of years with repeated chest X rays have shown disappearance of stage 1 or 2 nodulation with the development of panlobular emphysema. This progression poses problems for the diagnosis of CWP if these cases are not examined before the development of emphysema. The comparatively rare variety of "giant bullous emphysema" has been observed with unusual frequency in miners, even in those who do not smoke cigarettes, and this may represent a special complication of pneumoconiosis (32). The progression of other types of chronic diffuse pulmonary infiltration to emphysema has been well described (33). In the same way, it is possible that emphysema may be a common complication of the fibrosis due to CWP.

REFERENCES

1. Lieben, J., Pendergrass, E. G., and McBride, W. W. (1961). *J. Occup. Med.* **3**, 493.
2. McBride, W. W., Pendergrass, E. G., and Lieben, J. (1963). *J. Occup. Med.* **5**, 376.
3. McBride, W. W., Pendergrass, E. G., and Lieben, J. (1966). *J. Occup. Med.* **8**, 365.
4. Morgan, W. K. C. (1968). *Amer. Rev. Resp. Dis.* **98**, 306.
5. Rogan, J. M. (1963). "Annual Report for the Year 1963." Med. Ser. Med. Res., Nat. Coal Board, London.
6. Hart, J. R., Cochrane, A. L., and Higgins, I. T. T. (1963). *Tubercle* **44**, 141.
7. Browne, R. C. (1966). "The Chemistry and Therapy of Industrial Pulmonary Diseases." Thomas, Springfield, Illinois.
8. Nagelschmidt, G., *et al.* (1963). *Brit. J. Ind. Med.* **20**, 181.
9. Fallon, J. T. (1937). *Can. Med. Ass. J.* **36**, 223.
10. Vigliani, E. C., and Pernis, B. (1958). *Brit. J. Ind. Med.* **15**, 8.
11. Caplan, A. (1953). *Thorax* **8**, 29.
12. Caplan, A., Payne, R. B., and Withey, J. L. (1962). *Thorax* **17**, 205.
13. Gough, J. (1959). "Proceedings of the Pneumoconiosis Conference, Johannesburg, 1959" (A. J. Orenstein, ed.). Little, Brown, Boston, Mass.
14. Bramwell, B. (1914). *Edinburgh Med. J.* **12**, 387.
15. Erasmus, L. D. (1959). "Proceedings of the Pneumoconiosis Conference, Johannesburg, 1959" (A. G. Orenstein, ed.). Little, Brown, Boston, Mass.
16. Rodman, G. P., *et al.* (1967). *Ann. Int. Med.* **66**, 323.
17. Vigliani, E. C., and Pernis, B. (1963). *Advan. Tuberc. Res.* **12**, 230.
18. Fishman, A. P. (1961). *Physiol. Rev.* **41**, 214.
19. Lavenne, F. (1959). "Proceedings of the Pneumoconiosis Conference, Johannesburg, 1959" (A. J. Orenstein, ed.). Little, Brown, Boston, Mass.
20. Rasmussen, D. L., *et al.* (1968). *Amer. Rev. Resp. Dis.* **98**, 658.
21. Petty, T. L., *et al.* (1965). *Amer. Rev. Resp. Dis.* **92**, 450.
22. Colp, C., Park, S. S., and Williams, M. H., Jr. (1970). *Amer. Rev. Resp. Dis.* **101**, 615.
23. Penman, R. W. B., O'Neill, R. P., and Begley, L. (1970). *Amer. Rev. Resp. Dis.* **101**, 528.
24. Penman, R. W. B., O'Neill, R. P., and Begley, L. (1970). *Amer. Rev. Resp. Dis.* **101**, 536.
25. American Thoracic Society, Committee on Diagnostic Standards for Non-Tuberculous Respiratory Disease (1902). *Amer. Rev. Resp. Dis.* **85**, 762.
26. World Health Organization (1961). "Definitions and Diagnosis of Pulmonary Diseases with Special Reference to Chronic Bronchitis and Emphysema, *in* Chronic Cor Pulmonale." *World Health Organ. Tech. Rep. Ser.* **213**, 15.
27. Fletcher, C. M. (ed.) (1959). *Thorax* **14**, 286.
28. Heppleston, A. G. (1953). *J. Pathol. Bacteriol.* **66**, 235.
29. Heppleston, A. G. (1955). *Lab. Invest.* **4**, 374.
30. Leopold, J. G., and Gough, J. (1957). *Thorax* **12**, 219.
31. Sutinen, S., *et al.* (1965). *Amer. Rev. Resp. Dis.* **91**, 69.
32. O'Neill, R. P. (1970). Unpublished communication.
33. Cullen, J. H., Katy, H. C., and Kaemmerlen, J. T. (1965). *Amer. Rev. Resp. Dis.* **92**, 775.

PART 3
TREATMENT AND CONTROL

10

Etiology

Douglas H. K. Lee

Coal workers' pneumoconiosis is commonly defined as a diagnosable disorder of the respiratory system occurring in persons exposed to coal dust and presumably attributable to its inhalation. Implicit in the descriptions of symptoms, clinical manifestations, radiographic changes, and pathology described in some detail in the preceding chapters has been an acceptance of the above definition and of what might be called the gross etiological picture. But even at the gross level, this and similar definitions leave one with an uncomfortable feeling of being presented with a platitude or at least a circular argument—coal workers' pneumoconiosis is pneumoconiosis in a (identified) coal worker.

The term *pneumoconiosis* in the definition implicates dust, and presumably coal dust, as the prime etiologic agent, but it makes no commitment on the composition of the dust, on what component is responsible, or on what concomitant conditions of exposure may be playing a role. Nor does it answer an awkward hypothetical question—What would be the diagnosis of an identical condition in a person for whom exposure to coal dust is denied? (It is instructive to note in passing that coal workers' pneumoconiosis is not alone in this diagnostic dilemma. Byssinosis, baggasosis, and berylliosis involve similarly pragmatic and probabilistic diagnoses, depending, at least antemortem, upon a declared history of exposure rather than on an objectively demonstrable agent.) The etiology of coal workers' pneumoconiosis clearly deserves deeper study.

Role of Coal Dust

That respiratory disorders are closely associated with exposure to coal dust, and particularly dust occurring in the mining of coal, was progressively established over the last century as revealed by the writings of Meiklejohn (1, 2), Rosen (3), Sayers and colleagues (4, 5), Levine and Hunter (6), Lieben and colleagues (7–9), Lainhart *et al.* (10, 11), and others listed in a Public Health Service bibliography (12). (See Chapter 1.) Among the more telling recent pieces of evidence are:

The experience of the National Coal Board of Great Britain that the prevalence of radiographic changes increases with the prevailing concentration of dust in the mine air (13)

General absence of progress in radiographic changes if the miner is removed from exposure before stage 2 or PMF appears (13)

Relationship between the weight and composition of lung dust as seen postmortem and in radiographic findings (14, 15)

Relationship between occurrence of pulmonary changes and cumulative dust exposure in Ruhr Colliery studies (16)

Decreased certification rate, decreased age–specific prevalence of simple pneumoconiosis, and decreased overall prevalence of pneumoconiotic changes in British miners following the establishment of a limit of allowable dust concentration in 1949 (17, 18)

That the coal in the dust can serve as the etiologic agent, apart from other components such as silica or hydrocarbons, or ancillary factors such as smoking, is strongly suggested by several pieces of evidence, and particularly by the following:

The appearance of pneumoconiotic changes in coal trimmers (men shoveling coal in ships' bunkers to preserve the trim) who were working with coal from which country rock had been washed (19) and by the absence of unusual quantities of silica in their lungs at autopsy (20)

The development of pneumoconiosis roentgenographically and pathologically similar to coal workers' pneumoconiosis in persons exposed to natural graphite that contained very little free silica (21), to silica-free carbon (22), or to activated charcoal dust (23)

Poor correlation between the development of pneumoconiosis in British coal miners and the silica content of the mine rock (24)

Differences between the histopathology of the coal macule characteristic of coal workers' pneumoconiosis and that of the typical silicotic lesion—(a) in being peribronchiolar instead of interstitial; (b) in lacking the redundant fibrotic reaction with formation of typical whorls; and (c) in having low silica content (13)

The low concentration of silica in both Appalachian and European coal miners' lungs, seldom greatly exceeding the normal concentration of 200 mg/100 g of dried lung, as compared with the concentration of coal which constitutes 80% of the total dust present (13)

Role of Other Factors

In actual practice, of course, miners are exposed to a variety of other agents and conditions at the same time they inhale coal dust, many of which can affect respiratory function and integrity. The exact role that coal dust per se plays in the disease state exhibited by an individual probably varies very greatly with the particular mix of agents and conditions to which he has been exposed and, of course, with his own physiological constitution. To the extent that a responsive animal experimental model can be developed, an indication of the relative synergistic or modifying effect of important concurrent factors on the basic reactions to coal dust as such could be elucidated. For the present, one accepts the evidence cited above for coal as a primary etiologic agent and tries to estimate from epidemiologic and clinicopathologic evidence the extent to which these other factors participate as well and to which they should therefore be considered for control.

OCCUPATIONAL FACTORS

Silica occurs to varying extent in the country rock. A certain amount is likely to be included in the coal cut from the seam, and its dust is added to the mine air. Miners engaged in rock drilling, as opposed to coal getting, are exposed to stone dust to a greater extent, and it was these workers who exhibited the most pronounced effects among nineteenth century British miners. (See also Chapter 6, p. 107.) The extensive use of sand for traction on the rails in the haulage ways of United States coal mines and the recent increase in "roof-bolting" where the drilling may be very dusty may also increase the opportunity for silica dust as well as coal dust to have its effect (25). In a recent survey of 29 major mines conducted by the Bureau of Mines, the free silica content of "essentially coal mine dust" averaged around 2%, and in no case exceeded 3.5% (26). (See also Chapter 2, p. 22 and Table IV.)

Fumes from explosives and from burning electric cables contain various hydrocarbons and nitrogen oxides. Gases of this nature have been incriminated in the production of pulmonary diseases such as bronchitis and lung cancer in persons other than miners. The bronchitic effects may certainly exacerbate those accompanying pneumoconiosis, but fumes are unlikely to play any important role in the pneumoconiosis itself. Carcinogenesis is a separate pathological process which is apparently no more common among coal miners than among nonmining groups with similar smoking habits.

NONOCCUPATIONAL FACTORS

The synergistic role of *cigarette smoking* in facilitating pulmonary reactions to other agents is becoming increasingly clear. A dramatic case has been made for its effect on the incidence of bronchial carcinoma in asbestos workers (27), and evidence indicates a similar, although less marked, effect in uranium miners (28). Cigarette consumption by coal miners seems to be not very different from that of nonminers, in spite of the restrictions of underground working. Rasmussen found the reduction of ventilatory capacity and the increase in both residual volume and end alveolar nitrogen after 7 minutes of oxygen breathing in coal miners closely related to the heaviness of smoking (13). Hyatt and colleagues (29) showed much the same effect in a survey of 287 miners in West Virginia. The effect of smoking in coal miners is presumably one of facilitating secondary effects such as bronchitis and emphysema rather that of participation in the genesis of the initial macule. Smoking's role here seems to be a little different from that played in the production of bronchogenic carcinoma.

Climatic conditions, particularly those of Appalachian winters, may do something to facilitate infection and aggravate any preexisting bronchitis in miners emerging from warm underground conditions. They may add their quota to the clinical picture, but in secondary fashion.

Air pollution from industrial processes or from burning culm piles, that depressing feature of an erstwhile attractive scene, can undoubtedly add to the symptomatology of miners already suffering from bronchitis and emphysema. Pollution may accentuate and perhaps accelerate secondary pathological processes; however, it is unlikely to play any important part in the causation of the initial lesions.

Poor nutrition, substandard housing, and *depressed social conditions* probably reduce systemic resistance to environmental insults in those who are thus disadvantaged, rendering immune and compensatory responses less effective at all stages of the disease and increasing the opportunity for infection to be superimposed.

INFECTIVE FACTORS

Chronic bronchitis notoriously results from the interactive effects of several factors, predominant among which is infection with a variety of nonspecific organisms. The chronic bronchitis so often seen in those afflicted with pneumoconiosis is no exception. The two-thirds of the day spent away from the mine provides at least as much opportunity for infection to occur as does the mine environment itself.

The role of the *tuberculosis* organism (*Mycobacterium tuberculosis*) is not so clear. The lesions of progressive massive fibrosis in many ways resemble those of tuberculous infection in silicotic lungs, but the incidence of identifiable mycobacteria is less in those with PMF than those with classical silicosis, and many of those found appear atypical. Sputum from patients with PMF seldom induces tuberculosis in test guinea pigs, but recovery of organisms is not frequent even in cases of tuberculous silicosis. Belief in the tuberculosis organism as the prime cause of PMF changes is now less than it was 15 years ago, and its role in uncomplicated pneumoconiosis is virtually dismissed. As the result of a marked reduction in the prevalence of pulmonary tuberculosis in the general population, the opportunities for infection of coal miners have dwindled to the point where the organism is no longer regarded as an important factor, even under the less than satisfactory living conditions of many coal communities, but the incidence of PMF in coal miners does not appear to have been reduced in like measure. (See also Chapter 9, p. 182.)

CONSTITUTIONAL FACTORS

The degree of pathological response to coal dust among persons having presumably comparable exposures can vary greatly. The nature of individual variation in ability to deal with the inhaled dust is not known. Differences may be postulated in the patency of airways, the number of lung lobules utilized, macrophagic activity, immune responses, disposition of dust particles, resistance of arterioles to occlusion, and a host of other biological responses.

The persons making up a coal community, and particularly those of long standing, have been subjected to considerable selection by economic and traditional factors. It is possible that there may have been some concentration of genetic deficiencies in such critical items as the alpha-1 antitrypsin factor, without which an individual would be predisposed to an emphysematous response to a condition threatening the integrity of the lung alveoli (30). But until an adequate survey is made of such deficiencies in coal mining populations, the idea is purely speculative and can be given no particular credence in the etiology.

A more probable reason for varied response to dust may lie in variation in individual breathing habits, such as the volume of air respired for a given level of work, the depth and rate of respiration, postural limitations on lung expansion, and efficiency in use of rest periods. The cumulative result of such habit differences could be quite important over a period in excess of 20 years, but we are getting into individual variations about a common etiology rather than the etiology itself, whose central features may now be summarized.

Conclusions

The group of respiratory disturbances occurring in coal miners that are subsumed under the nosological term "coal workers' pneumoconiosis" is primarily due to the inhalation of coal dust. In practice, however, the picture is usually complicated by the simultaneous operation of several other factors which may modify the symptomatology, pathology, and clinical course of the disease. Prominent among these are such occupational factors as silica dust, nonoccupational factors such as cigarette smoking, various infective factors such as the numerous nonspecific organisms found in bronchitic lesions, and individual variability of pulmonary response and resistance to stress. The dividing line between cases of respiratory disease in which coal dust plays some role and those in which coal dust is innocent of effect is virtually impossible to define. (See Chapter 3, p. 29.)

The gross etiological association of respiratory diseases in coal miners with exposure to coal dust provides the basis for attempting to control their incidence by reducing the concentrations of dust to which coal miners are exposed. It also provides the basis on which measures for compensation of affected coal miners may be considered.

Refinement of the etiological picture involves establishing the nature and extent of the role played by factors other than coal dust in the initiation and development of the pleomorphic disease picture. The knowledge so gained would indicate the extent to which etiologic factors other than coal dust should also be controlled in the interests of reducing the incidence or the progress of the disease. It also would contribute to a better understanding of pulmonary reactions to environmental insults of various kinds and establish the features of pulmonary pathology that these diseases share with reactions to other environmental threats.

ACKNOWLEDGMENTS

In preparing this chapter the author has drawn heavily from the sources mentioned in Chapter 1, and also from the views expressed at a small symposium held at NIEHS in June 1969 (13), but takes full responsibility for the conclusions expressed here.

REFERENCES

1. Meiklejohn, A. (1951). *Brit. J. Ind. Med.* **8**, 127.
2. Meiklejohn, A. (1962). *Brit. J. Ind. Med.* **9**, 93, 208.
3. Rosen, G. (1943). "History of Miners' Diseases." Schuman, New York.
4. Sayers, R. R., *et al.* (1934). *Pa. Dept. Labor Industry, Spec. Bull.* 41.
5. Sayers, R. R., *et al.* (1935). *U. S. Pub. Health Bull.* 221.
6. Levine, M. D., and Hunter, M. B. (1957). *J. Amer. Med. Ass.* **163**, 1.
7. Lieben, J., Pendergrass, E., and McBride, W. W. (1961). *J. Occup. Med.* **3**, 493.
8. Lieben, J., and Hill, P. C. (1962). *Pa. Med. J.* **65**, 1475.
9. Lieben, J. (1967). "Coal Miners' Pneumoconiosis in Pennsylvania—1967." *W. Va. School Med. Centen. Symp. Coal Workers' Pneumoconiosis.*
10. Lainhart, W. S., *et al.* (1968). *Arch. Environ. Health* **16**, 207.
11. Lainhart, W. S., *et al.* (1969). "Pneumoconiosis in Appalachian Bituminous Coal Miners." Govt. Print. Off., Washington, D. C.
12. Doyle, H. N., and Noehren, T. H. (1954). *U. S. Pub. Health Bibliogr. Ser.* 11.
13. Lee, D. H. K. (1971). "Coal Workers' Pneumoconiosis—State of Knowledge and Research Needs." *J. Occup. Med.* (in press).
14. Rivers, D., *et al.* (1960). *Brit. J. Ind. Med.* **17**, 87.
15. Rossiter, E. C., *et al.* (1965). *Brit. Occup. Hyg. Soc. Symp.*, Paper 64.
16. Reisner, J. (1968). *Beitr. Silikose. Forsch.* **95**, 1.
17. National Coal Board (1969). *Med. Ser. Med. Res. Ann. Rep. 1967–1968.*
18. National Coal Board (1968). "Report and Accounts 1967–68. I. Report." HMSO, London.
19. Collis, E. L., and Gilchrist, J. C. (1928). *J. Ind. Hyg.* **10**, 101.
20. Gough, J. (1940). *J. Pathol. Bacteriol.* **51**, 277.
21. Watson, A. J., *et al.* (1959). *Brit. J. Ind. Med.* **16**, 274.
22. Gaensler, E. A., *et al.* (1966). *Amer. J. Med.* **41**, 864.
23. Lainhart, W. S., and Cralley, L. J., unpublished data.
24. Nagelschmidt, G. (1965). *Amer. J. Ind. Hyg. Ass.* **26**, 1.
25. Kerr, L. E. (1956). *Ind. Med. Surg.* **25**, 355.
26. "Papers and Proceedings of the National Conference on Medicine and the Federal Coal Mine Health and Safety Act of 1969" (1970). Washington, D. C.
27. Selikoff, I. J., Hammond, E. C., and Churg, J. (1968). *J. Amer. Med. Ass.* **204**, 106.
28. Lundin, F. E., *et al.* (1969). *Health Phys.* **16**, 571.
29. Hyatt, R. E., Kisten, A. D., and Mahan, T. K. (1963). *Amer. Rev. Resp. Dis.* **89**, 387.
30. Resnick, H., Lapp, N. L., and Morgan, W. K. C. (1971). *J. Amer. Med. Ass.* **215**, 1101.

11

Treatment

Leon Cander

The basis of all rational therapy, whether specific or symptomatic, is accurate diagnosis. Because of the controversy surrounding the diagnosis of coal workers' pneumoconiosis as well as the medicolegal implications of the diagnosis, it might be well to spend a few moments considering certain aspects of the diagnosis of CWP.

Let us begin by accepting the fact that the inhalation of coal dust alone can produce serious, chronic, disabling disease of the lungs. Although Part 410 of the Federal Coal Mine Health and Safety Act of 1969, Public Law 91-173 (1), requires some form of dust opacification on the chest X ray for the diagnosis of CWP during life, several recent reports (2, 3) indicate the presence of significant pulmonary insufficiency involving primarily ventilation/perfusion inequalities and abnormal alveolar gas exchange as well as pulmonary disability in coal miners with normal chest X rays. Similar findings have been reported in patients with chronic bronchitis and bronchial asthma (4). These studies simply underscore the often observed lack of correlation between X-ray findings, pulmonary function tests, and pulmonary disability in all chronic intrinsic disease of the lungs (5). Rasmussen's findings (2, 3) suggest that the X-ray requirement of Public Law 91-173 may be too stringent, thereby excluding a number of miners disabled by CWP. This statement is not a criticism of Public Law 91-173, which is a landmark in legislation—it is simply a recognition of the need for more precise diagnostic criteria for CWP.

While *pulmonary insufficiency* refers to an abnormality of lung function demonstrable by objective physiologic techniques, *pulmonary disability* refers to decreased working capacity owing to the disease state. Of interest in the studies referred to above (2–4) is the demonstration of normal values for routine pulmonary function tests, especially those used to assess ventilatory capacity, in the presence of significant degrees of dyspnea (disability). It was only by the use of more sophisticated methods which assessed the functioning of peripheral airways and distal ramifications of the pulmonary arteries that significant degrees of pulmonary insufficiency were documented. These studies reveal the similarities of disturbed lung function in CWP and nonspecific chronic obstructive lung disease. They also highlight the need for continued longitudinal research on patients to obtain a better understanding of the natural history of CWP as well as a more precise picture of the disordered physiology and its possible relationship to pulmonary disability. Such data will permit a more just evaluation of disability associated with CWP and form the basis for an even more rational management of the disease. Data thus derived should also permit quantitation of the degree of disability and establishment of a scale of compensation to supplant the present all-or-none regulation of Public Law 91-173.

Because of the lack of longitudinal studies on patients with CWP in our country, many aspects of the natural history of CWP are largely unknown. Hence, assessment of the results of any therapy is extremely difficult. Ever since Rudolf von Virchow, physicians have known that anatomic alterations in organs and tissues produced by disease result in disturbed function. When the anatomic alteration is permanent, then the functional derangement is also permanent unless compensatory mechanisms can restore function to the normal state. Available evidence indicates that the fundamental anatomic lesion in CWP, the coal macule, leads to organization and fibrous scarring resulting from the presence of coal dust in the lung. With time, the scars shrink, leading to distortion of the lung structures. Thus there is every reason to believe that once established, the fundamental disease process cannot be completely arrested in CWP. There is evidence to support this view (6, 7). Because no known therapy can arrest or reverse the disease process, the major thrust today is in preventive medicine. Consideration should be given to removing from a dusty working atmosphere any miner whose lung function shows rapid deterioration or whose X ray reveals unusually rapid progression. Similarly, because of the high attack rate of progressive massive fibrosis among miners with category 3, simple pneumoconiosis [ILO classification (8)], this group should be removed from any mining job where there is a high concentration of respirable coal dust. That part of Public Law 91-173 which sets limits on the concentration of respirable dust in coal mines is the most powerful weapon available today for preventing the development of disabling CWP in coal miners. It has been shown that effective dust suppression in the mines reduces the incidence of CWP (9).

General Aspects

At the present time treatment of patients with CWP is symptomatic and indicated only when cough, sputum, wheezing, and dyspnea are present. Certain respiratory and nonrespiratory complications occur with increased frequency in these patients and deserve comment. These complications include infected bronchitis, acute pulmonocardiac failure, cor pulmonale with congestive heart failure, pulmonary tuberculosis, and peptic ulcer. It should be noted that asymptomatic, uncomplicated CWP requires no therapy other than reassurance.

Before initiating a therapeutic program, it is important to explain the nature of the disease process to the patient, dispelling any fears and securing his cooperation in a long-term program on a note of cautious optimism. In terms of management, the patient with CWP uncomplicated by any of the conditions listed above may be viewed as someone with chronic obstructive lung disease; only reversible bronchial obstruction will respond to treatment. Poor advice could be more disabling than the disease. As with any chronic disease, both patient and physician must have limited, realistic objectives as goals of therapy. These goals are (1) relief of bronchial obstruction, improvement of ventilation and reduction of the work of breathing, and (2) a program of physical activity and employment consistent with the degree of pulmonary disability. Since weight gain has a deleterious effect on lung function (10), if physical activity must be reduced, then an appropriate reduction in caloric intake should be made to prevent weight gain.

A point worth emphasis is the absolute necessity for patients who are symptomatic from CWP to stop smoking cigarettes. The relationship between cigarette smoking and the presence of chronic bronchitis and emphysema has been established beyond a doubt and deserves little comment here. Whether cigarette smoking potentiates the effects of the inhaled coal dust or is synergistic is unknown; what is known is that the effects of cigarette smoking and inhaled coal dust are greater than the effect of either alone (11), and either alone can produce serious, chronic, disabling pulmonary disease. Continued cigarette smoking will nullify the effect of any therapy used to provide symptomatic relief and will hasten the development of disabling disease. In fact, it would be well if all coal miners were to stop smoking cigarettes.

RELIEF OF BRONCHIAL OBSTRUCTION

The reduction of sputum viscosity by steam inhalation and a fluid intake of at least 3 liters/day will increase the efficacy of postural drainage in removing excessive secretions. Bronchodilator drugs will alleviate to some extent any reversible bronchial obstruction. Objective assessment of the response to bronchodilator drugs by noting any improvement in such simple tests as the midmaximal flow rate is the most certain guide to therapy. Bronchodilator agents should be administered both locally by aerosol (e.g., isoproterenol 1:200) and systemically (ephedrine sulphate by mouth and aqueous aminophylline instilled rectally) since parts of the lung which are completely occluded will not be reached by aerosols. Because of the high incidence of induced cardiac arrhythmias, the frequency of inhalation of sympathomimetic amine aerosols should be limited.

IMPROVEMENT OF VENTILATION

Over the past few decades many procedures have been suggested to improve alveolar ventilation in patients with bronchoobstructive disease. However, no method has met with uniform success. Breathing exercises are of questionable value according to evidence obtained from lung function testing (12). However, they may be employed for their psychological value. Drugs which depress the central nervous system (e.g., narcotics, sedatives, tranquilizers) should not be used in these patients. These agents cause alveolar hypoventilation, suppress the cough reflex, and lead to retention of secretions, increasing the physiologic derangement and defeating the aims of therapy.

Complications

ACUTE BRONCHITIS

All patients should be put to bed to minimize metabolic demands on an already compromised ventilatory apparatus. Antibiotics are not indicated for most acute respiratory infections because of their viral etiology. Microscopic (Gram stain) and bacteriologic examination should be carried out on all patients. If the sputum is purulent and the predominant organism is a gram-positive coccus, therapy may be initiated (pending the laboratory report) with 400,000 units of intramuscular aqueous penicillin every 6 hours. Alternatively, if the predominant organism is a gram-negative bacillus, or there is a mixed infection, therapy may be initiated with 250 mg of ampicillin by mouth every six hours. Changes in antibiotic therapy should be dictated by the results of in vitro sensitivity tests. Antibiotic therapy should be continued for at least one week following clinical improvement and reduction of pus cells and bacteria in the sputum. Because of the danger of induced aplastic anemia, chloramphenicol should be employed only in life-threatening situations.

Hydration should be maintained and bronchodilator therapy intensified throughout the period of acute infection.

ACUTE PULMONOCARDIAC FAILURE

Simultaneous occurrence of acute pulmonary and myocardial failure is usually induced by an acute respiratory infection. This situation may also be precipitated by oxygen administration, spontaneous pneumothorax, depressant drugs, or surgery. All of the precipitating causes result in a further reduction in alveolar ventilation and a rise in arterial carbon dioxide tension with its attendant central nervous system depression and coma (carbon dioxide narcosis). Hospitalization is imperative in this medical emergency. These patients require intensive care.

Details of management of this life-threatening situation have been covered in a recent publication to which the reader is referred (13).

COR PULMONALE AND CONGESTIVE HEART FAILURE

In view of the high incidence of cor pulmonale in patients with CWP, especially bituminous miners, congestive heart failure is an all too common complication in miners past the age of 50 (14). Unfortunately, the diagnosis of cor pulmonale can only be established clinically when the process is usually too well established to be reversible.

Patients with congestive heart failure should be hospitalized. Since the majority of these patients are hypoxic in the presence of hyperventilation, oxygen should be administered without the fear of inducing hypercapnia. Arterial blood gas tensions should be measured frequently for monitoring. Raising the arterial oxygen tension is essential if maximum effect from digitalis and diuretic therapy is to be achieved. Owing to the frequency with which digitalis toxicity occurs in these patients, digitalization should be accomplished slowly and cautiously over 3–4 days. The end point of digitalization is rarely clear-cut, and the first evidence of digitalis toxicity may be a supraventricular tachycardia, especially paroxysmal atrial tachycardia with block. For these reasons, if available, continuous EKG monitoring should be employed during digitalization.

Because of the frequency with which serious cardiac arrhythmias occur in this situation, diuretic agents should be used cautiously, accompanied by frequent determinations of the serum potassium concentration. Sodium restriction and bed rest should be employed to meet the needs of the patient.

PULMONARY TUBERCULOSIS

It has been demonstrated that chemotherapy has no beneficial effect on patients with sputum-negative, early complicated pneumoconiosis (15). It would seem at the present that there is no place for antituberculous chemoprophylaxis in sputum-negative patients with CWP.

Although it has been shown that the presence of CWP diminishes the response to chemotherapy in patients with sputum-positive tuberculosis, triple therapy (isonicotinic acid hydrazide, streptomycin, and para-amino-salicylic acid), when continued for at least 2 and preferably 3 years, will convert the majority of patients (16). It is essential that drug sensitivities be determined on all patients to provide the surest guide to effective chemotherapy. This is of even greater importance in patients who have received prior chemotherapy.

PEPTIC ULCER

Patients with CWP, as is true of patients with chronic bronchitis and emphysema, manifest an increased incidence of peptic ulcer (17). Because of the unusually high rate of occurrence of active pulmonary tuberculosis and progressive massive fibrosis following partial gastrectomy in patients with CWP, it is recommended that surgery be avoided, if at all possible, in the treatment of peptic ulcer in these patients (18).

REFERENCES

1. Part 410—Federal Coal Mine Health and Safety Act of 1969, Title IV—"Black Lung Benefits" (1970). *Fed. Regist.* **35**, 5623 (No. 67).
2. Rasmussen, D. L., *et al.* (1968). *Amer. Rev. Resp. Dis.* **98**, 658.
3. Rasmussen, D. L. (1970). "Impairment of Oxygen Transfer in Dyspneic, Non-Smoking Soft Coal Miners from Southern Appalachian Coal Fields," *in* Papers and Proceedings of the National Conference on Medicine and the Federal Coal Mine Health and Safety Act of 1969, Washington, D. C.
4. Levine, G., *et al.* (1970). *New Eng. J. Med.* **282**, 1277.
5. Hunter, D. (1969). "The Diseases of Occupation." Little, Brown, Boston, Mass.
6. Duguid, J. B., and Lambert, M. W. (1964). *J. Pathol. Bacteriol.* **88**, 389.
7. Coni, N. K. (1967). *Brit. J. Ind. Med.* **24**, 243.
8. Cochrane, A. L. (1962). *Brit. J. Ind. Med.* **19**, 52.
9. Hendricks, Ch. A. M., and Claus, H. (1963). *Brit. J. Ind. Med.* **20**, 288.
10. Cotes, J. E., and Gilson, J. C. (1967). *Ann. Occup. Hyg.* **10**, 327.
11. Tokuhata, G. K., *et al.* (1970). *Amer. J. Pub. Health* **60**, 441.
12. Campbell, E. J. M., and Friend, J. (1955). *Lancet* **1**, 325.
13. Cander, L. (1970). *In* "Pre- and Postoperative Management of the Cardiopulmonary Patient." Grune and Stratton, New York.
14. Naeye, R. L. (1970). "Soft Coal Workers' Pneumoconiosis—A Quantitative,

Post-Mortem Study," *in* Papers and Proceedings of the National Conference on Medicine and the Federal Coal Mine and Health Safety Act of 1969, Washington, D. C.
15. Ball, J. D., *et al.* (1969). *Thorax* **24**, 399.
16. Joint Investigators of the Medical Research Council (1967). *Tubercle* **48**, 1.
17. Schwartz, R. (1970). "Non-Respiratory Illnesses of Coal Miners," in Papers and Proceedings of the National Conference on Medicine and the Federal Coal Mine and Safety Act of 1969, Washington, D. C.
18. Phillips, T. J. G. (1970). *Brit. J. Ind. Med.* **27**, 245.

12

Investigations in Progress

BIOMEDICAL

W. Keith C. Morgan and Earle P. Shoub

Although much is currently known about coal workers' pneumoconiosis, there are still many gaping voids in our knowledge. Thus although the inhalation of coal dust is essential to the development of this disease, a linear relationship between dust exposure and the development and progression of CWP is often not evident. There remain many unexplained anomalies, and much still remains to be done. The U. S. Public Health Service is currently involved in a number of studies which it is hoped will shed light on some of these mysteries. The more important of these are worth description.

National (Inter-Agency) Study of Coal Workers' Pneumoconiosis

In both Great Britain and Germany, long-term prospective studies attempting to relate the development and progression of coal workers' pneumoconiosis to the levels of dust prevailing in the coal mines have been in progress for many years. Workers from both countries presented their data at the Third International Conference on Inhaled Particles in London in September 1970, and the similarity of their findings, considering their varied methodology, was quite remarkable (1, 2). While the British use gravimetric sampling to measure respirable dust concentrations, the Germans use the Tyndalloscope. Despite this and other differences, the projected attack rates for given concentrations of dust were very similar.

In late 1968, it became apparent that no comparable prospective study was being carried out in the United States, and therefore, the U. S. Public Health Service and Bureau of Mines decided to remedy this deficiency by devising a similar study for coal mines in the United States. The data accumulated by the British and German workers have formed the basis for the permissible dust levels in their respective coal mines. Lacking comparable data here, it was realized that any health standards in the United States would have to be based on work carried out elsewhere.

The National Study of Coal Workers' Pneumoconiosis (Inter-Agency Study) is a joint effort of the Bureau of Mines and the Public Health Service. Over 30 coal mines in various parts of the United States have been selected for inclusion in the study. The criteria for selection were that the mines should have at least 100 miners, that they should have an estimated working life of at least 10, but preferably more years, that they should represent all the geographical areas of the United States in which coal mining remains a major industry, that different seams of coal with differing ranks and mineral content should be included, and finally that the mining methods used in the various mines should be diverse. The mines chosen for inclusion in the study are to be found in the following States: Pennsylvania, West Virginia, Virginia, Alabama, Tennessee, Kentucky, Ohio, Illinois, Indiana, Utah, and Colorado. It is expected that some 7500 to 8000 miners will be included; moreover, it is hoped to extend the study in the future. Up to now some 5000 active coal miners from Pennsylvania and West Virginia have been examined.

All the men employed in the selected mines either have been or will be asked to undergo a medical examination. This consists of a posteroanterior and left lateral chest film and some simple tests of ventilatory capacity. In addition, a questionnaire concerning the presence of cough, sputum, and shortness of breath is administered. A detailed smoking and occupational history is taken. Anthropometric measurements are made, and the subject is then asked to perform three forced vital capacity (FVC) maneuvers. Prior to the measurements being recorded, he is given two trial runs so that he understands what is required. The respiratory maneuvers are recorded as flow volume loops on a recording oscilloscope, and if all three appear satisfactory, they are photographed with a Polaroid camera. From the loop, the FEV_1, $FEV_{0.75}$, FVC, peak flow, and midflow are recorded. From the posteroanterior and lateral film, the total lung capacity (TLC) is measured and the residual volume (RV) is derived by subtracting the FVC from the TLC.

The medical examinations will be repeated at intervals of 5 years except on the first occasion when there will be only a 3-year interval. Comparison of the chest films taken at each examination will allow the Public Health Service to determine radiological progression over this period. In addition, repetition of the pulmonary function tests will determine the annual decrement in ventilatory capacity over the same period. This can then be related to the presence or absence of pneumoconiosis, to the miner's smoking habits, and to various other factors.

The Bureau of Mines will be responsible for environmental measurements in the selected coal mines. Levels of respirable dust will be determined by several different instruments, including the Mining Research Establishment (MRE) horizontal elutriator and the Atomic Energy Commission (AEC) cyclone (personal sampler). Data will be developed which will permit estimation of the respirable dust exposure of underground workers in terms of milligram-years. A sufficient number of dust samples will be analyzed to estimate the influence of total ash, total combustibles, and total and free silica on the development and progression of pneumoconiosis, and at least 1% of all dust samples obtained from each mine will be subjected to a complete mineralogical analysis. The main purpose of the study will be to relate the radiological progression of the disease to the respirable dust levels that prevailed in the mines over the study period. It is expected that a relationship between the radiological findings and the magnitude of exposure to coal dust will be evident. Nonetheless, the British experience suggests that other factors play a role in the production of the disease, viz. the rank and mineral content of the coal mined, individual susceptibility of the exposed miners, and possibly the silica content of the coal (3). The relative importance of these factors should become more evident as the study progresses. The data accumulated should allow derivation of mathematical equations that predict the likelihood of men developing the various categories of the disease at differing levels of dust exposure for various periods. It is doubtful, however, that any sort of mathematical inferences of this type can be drawn with any certainty until an 8- to 10-year period has elapsed.

Studies of the Pathology and Biochemistry

While it has been known for some time that there is a fairly good correlation between the coal dust content of the lungs and the radiological category, that is to say, the more the dust, the higher the category, much debate is still taking place in regard to the material which is responsible for the radioopaque shadows seen in the chest film. In this context it is important to remember that carbon is nonopaque and does not cast a shadow. The Safety in Mines Research Establishment of Sheffield, England, has been carrying out a correlative study in which postmortem analyses of the lungs for various minerals and other agents, e.g., silica, iron, collagen, and coal are related to the antemortem radiographic appearances (4). They have shown that in addition to the correlation between radiological category and coal-dust content there exists an almost equally good relationship with the total mineral content of the lungs. The same applies to the iron content of the lung. However, the best relationship of all is found when the radiographic category is plotted against a composite scale based on the combined coal, mineral, and iron contents. Rather surprisingly, the Sheffield group has shown that the coal content of the lung in progressive massive fibrosis is of the same order as that found in categories-1 and -2 simple CWP.

No explanation is available for the different sized opacities (pinhead or p, micronodular or m, and nodular or n) that may be found in films of subjects with simple pneumoconiosis with the exception of the nodular (n) variety. The latter are sometimes related to the presence of rheumatoid factor in the serum, and many of these subjects have a variant of Caplan's syndrome. It is possible that the type of opacity found in the chest film varies with the coal, mineral, and iron content of the lungs, and needless to say, this is worth further consideration.

It is becoming apparent that there seem to be certain distinctive physiological abnormalities associated with the different types of opacity. Thus Lyons and his colleagues have reported that the pinhead type of opacity tends to be associated with a lower diffusing capacity (5). These findings have been confirmed in the Appalachian Laboratory for Occupational Respiratory Diseases (ALFORD). In addition, a few subjects with the pinhead opacity have been found to have mild pulmonary hypertension in the absence of any cause for it other than simple pneumoconiosis. There is a great need for studies designed to correlate changes in the various physiological indices with varying types of pulmonary opacity seen on the chest film. The reasons why irregular opacities predominate in certain films and why other films show only rounded regular opacities remain a mystery. It seems possible that the extent of focal emphysema or fibrosis may vary with the type of small opacity present in the lungs. Work along these lines is presently being carried on in ALFORD.

The pathological features of CWP are fairly well recognized, and the main argument today centers around the specificity of the bronchiolar dilatation or focal emphysema that is found in the center of the coal macule. This type of emphysema has been described in urban dwellers and is claimed by both Lynne Reid and Heard not to be specific for CWP. The other features of the coal macule seem to be well accepted, and most pathologists maintain that the pathology of CWP is the same the world over and that it is impossible to differentiate pathologically the lesion found in soft-coal workers from that found in anthracite miners, provided the latter have not developed classical silicosis from exposure to coal mine dust with a high silica content. When the quartz content of the total lung dust exceeds 18%, then the microscopic appearances are those of silicosis and not CWP. Yet despite the common histological features, epidemiological studies have shown wide regional differences in the prevalence of simple and complicated pneumoconiosis. Moreover, Heppleston has shown that dusts which have identical size and surface characteristics but are prepared from coals of different rank are treated differently in the lungs (6). There is a need for studies in which the deposition and clearance of various types of coal are characterized. In addition, the effects on biological systems of coal and other dusts that produce pneumoconiosis need to be studied. This can be best achieved by studying the action of the various dusts on tissue cultures of cells found in the lungs, e.g., macrophages and fibroblasts.

Many pneumoconioses are associated with changes in the laying down of the fibrous proteins of the lungs, viz. collagen, elastin, and reticulin. The factors governing the disposition of these proteins in the lungs of subjects with pneumoconiosis have barely been considered, and a fertile field exists for the interested biochemist. In this connection, the pathogenesis of progressive massive fibrosis still remains a matter of speculation despite the several theories put forward to explain its development. It is not known whether the disease is a single entity, and the recent demonstration that some subjects with PMF have rheumatoid factor in their serum and histological evidence of vasculitis in the conglomerate lesion raises the possibility that these subjects have an autoimmune process. Further evidence in favor of this hypothesis is the demonstration of lung autoantibodies in the serum of many of these subjects.

There is little doubt that the pathological process that leads to PMF starts long before the "one-centimeter" opacity becomes evident on the chest film. Attempts should be made to detect the lesion before it is evident on the chest film as a one-centimeter shadow. Were it possible to study the very early lesions by means of light and electron microscopy, some clues in regard to the pathogenesis of the condition might be found.

The factors that determine whether or not PMF progresses are of paramount importance, yet are completely unknown. The vast majority of subjects who develop PMF have small lesions which grow exceedingly slowly. In many instances, the lesion reaches a limited size and remains unchanged thereafter. A detailed study of the immunology and immunochemistry of subjects with PMF is likely to be rewarding in this regard.

Physiological Studies

The numerous epidemiological studies performed on coal miners have mostly relied on simple screening tests of pulmonary function, such as the forced expiratory volume in 1 second (FEV_1), or some other test derived from a forced vital capacity maneuver. While the normal inclination of the epidemiologist is to study large numbers of subjects inadequately, the physiologist studies a few subjects—usually the wrong ones—in meticulous detail. Somewhere between lies a happy medium which is hopefully represented by some of the current studies taking place in ALFORD.

Studies of Ventilation and Pulmonary Mechanics

It is commonly accepted that miners as a whole have a lower ventilatory capacity than do nonminers. The cause of this reduction remains a matter of speculation, however. Several hypotheses have been put forward to explain it. First, it has been suggested that the inhalation of dust by itself produces a form of chronic obstructive airway disease, and indeed there is some evidence that this is so. Nonetheless, the effects of cigarette smoking so outweigh all other factors in the production of bronchitis that confirmation of this theory is difficult. This problem can be approached by comparing the annual decrement in pulmonary function in nonsmoking miners with a similar group of nonminers. Another possible explanation for the low FEV_1 is related to coal miners having smoking habits different from the general male population. The miner smokes slightly fewer cigarettes than does his nonminer counterpart; however, he manages to do so in half the time since he is unable to smoke while underground. It is conceivable that the more intense insult is responsible. A third possible explanation is that of differential migration. Were the more fit miners more prone to leave the occupation of coal mining, then those who remain would be less fit and would probably have a lower ventilatory capacity and more symptoms. Finally, the possibility exists that the coal macule itself is responsible for the effect. The radiological appearance of CWP depends on the superimposition of numerous macules upon each other; yet it must be remembered that macroscopic macules are present in the lungs some time before they become radiologically evident. Relevant in this connection is the fact that airway resistance may be partitioned into central and peripheral components and that most of the resistance is to be found in the larger airways, the smaller airways being responsible for less than 20%. Yet the coal macule is peripherally situated and thus can only affect flow in the peripheral airways. It is, therefore, apparent that were 50% or even more of the distal airways obstructed, the total airway resistance would not be appreciably affected, and this would probably not be detected on conventional spirometry. The distensibility of the lung would, nevertheless, be changed to such an extent that the subject might well be short of breath. The resistance to flow in the peripheral airways can be studied by means of the expiratory flow volume loop and also by determination of the pulmonary compliance at different frequencies. Some indication of changes in the peripheral resistance also might be detected from a study of the full curve of airway resistance plotted against volume of thoracic gas. Finally there is a need for studies of static pressure volume curves of the coal miners' lungs to determine the possible presence of early lung destruction. All these studies are currently underway at ALFORD.

Studies of Gas Transfer and Diffusion

The reduced diffusing capacity found in United States coal miners with the pinhead type of simple pneumoconiosis has been mentioned elsewhere. There seems little doubt that this is a valid observation since the British and the Belgians have reported similar findings. This finding needs to be supplemented by further studies of oxygen and carbon dioxide exchange, especially during exercise, and the latter should be related to the presence of pulmonary disability. Additional studies of the pulmonary circulation are recommended in order to evaluate possible changes in the pulmonary capillary bed. These can be best effected by perfusion scans with radioactive iodinated human serum albumin. Radioactive xenon offers a sophisticated, but as yet unutilized approach to the investigation of ventilation perfusion abnormalities found in coal workers' pneumoconiosis.

REFERENCES

1. Jacobsen, M., *et al.* (in press). Proceedings of the 3rd International Symposium on Inhaled Particles, London, 1970.
2. Reisner, M. T. R. (1970). "Relationship between pneumoconiosis and dust exposure in British coal mines," presented at the Third International Symposium on Inhaled Particles, London.
3. Jacobsen, M., *et al.* (1970). *Nature* **227**, 445.
4. Rossiter, C. E., *et al.* (1967). Dust Content, Radiology, and Pathology in Simple Pneumoconiosis of Coalworkers *in* "Inhaled Particles and Vapours II," p. 419. Pergamon, New York.
5. Lyons, J. P., *et al.* (1967). *Brit. Med. J.* **4**, 772.
6. Heppelston, A. G. (1970). "Effects of duration and intermittency of exposure on the disposal of high and low rank coal in SPF rats," presented at the Third International Symposium on Inhaled Particles, London.

INSTRUMENTATION

Jeremiah R. Lynch

The exposure of coal miners to dust has traditionally been measured by impinger counting, as have most other industrial dust exposures. However, due to settling problems and lack of agreement between observers, the results obtained were of doubtful value. Research into the deposition and retention of inhaled particles led to the conclusion that a measurement based on the mass of respirable dust would be a more relevant index of risk of disease (1). Lippmann (2) had observed that a commercially available 10-mm nylon cyclone, developed originally for removing sand from water, when operated at a certain flow rate approximated the respirability criteria developed by the Atomic Energy Commission (AEC) for measurement of radioactive aerosols (3). In Britain, similar measurements were made with horizontal elutriators designed to approximate the Johannesburg criteria (4). Although the two instruments do not measure exactly the same dust fraction, they both provide a measure of the respirable fraction of dust. In the Federal Coal Mine Health and Safety Act of 1969 the British "MRE" horizontal elutriator was adopted as a standard, although "equivalent" instruments were permitted. Since the MRE is not suitable for measuring miner exposure, the majority of samples are being collected with the personal samplers based on a cyclone-type size-selective presampler.

Coal Mine Dust Personal Sampler

The coal mine dust personal sampling unit, as approved by the Bureau of Occupational Safety and Health under Title 30, Code of Federal Regulation, Part 74, 11 March 1970, consists of a 10-mm nylon cyclone connected to a cassette containing a preweighed filter capsule. Air is drawn through the sampling head by a rechargeable battery-powered pump attached to the miner's belt. Much of the work currently in progress is directed to the following factors which may affect the accuracy of the instrument:

Flow Rate. Several investigators have recommended different flow rates for approximating the AEC curve. At present a cyclone flow rate of 2.0 liters/minute is being used, and based on 1000 pairs of simultaneous MRE–cyclone samples, an equivalence of cyclone concentration $\times$ 1.6 = MRE concentration is used. A theoretical factor of about 1.25 should be obtained if both instruments are operating according to theory. Recent work has indicated that the cyclone flow rate should be 1.7 liters/minute, which will result in a lower equivalence factor. The exact empirical equivalence is being established based on simultaneous samples taken in coal mines at the new cyclone flow rate.

Flow Pulsation. All laboratory flow rate experiments have been performed using steady flow rates. In actual samplers the flow through the cyclone pulsates due to the action of the pump. This effect is being investigated so that either a correction of the flow rate or a pulsation dampener may be used to obtain the desired size-selective characteristics.

Particle Charge. The charge distribution found in real aerosols is different from that in laboratory-generated aerosols. Experiments are being performed to determine if wide variations in charge cause changes in cyclone performance.

Cyclone Orientation. The effect of orientation with respect to both ambient air currents and offsets from vertical is being considered.

Mass Loading. It is necessary to determine whether dust concentration or the total amount of dust retained affect cyclone performance either by reintrainment or changes in cyclone properties.

Particle Shape. It has been assumed that the separation obtained with a cyclone is uniquely described by the aerodynamic size of the particles. Some preliminary work suggests that particles with extreme shape factors may be passed or retained other than as predicted by their aerodynamic size.

In addition to evaluation of instrument variations, work is being done to evaluate the variability and characteristics of the coal mine dust environment for the purpose of developing improved sampling strategies.

The cyclone-type coal mine dust personal sampler was adopted because it was readily available and considerable work on its performance had already been done. It is by no means a perfect instrument, and much work is underway to investigate basic size-selective sampling methods leading to the development of a second-generation instrument intended specifically for respirable coal mine dust measurement.

Coal Mine Dust Monitoring Instruments

In addition to the investigation of instruments intended for determining compliance with respirable dust standards, a number of instruments are being developed for control or research purposes.

In order to evaluate the effectiveness of a particular control measure, it is desirable to be able to measure the instantaneous respirable coal mine dust concentration or at least to be able to make a measurement in a minute or less as opposed to many hours. Such data are also valuable for determining peak exposures in connection with toxicological research. Several principles are currently being investigated to develop such an "instantaneous" instrument:

Light Scattering. Light scattered from either single particles or clouds of particles may be detected by a photocell and read out as some measure of particle concentration. It is necessary to determine how such an index relates to respirable mass concentration.

Quartz Crystal. When dust is deposited on the surface of a quartz crystal, its natural resonant frequency is decreased. This change in frequency may be measured with considerable accuracy and related directly to particle mass. The extreme sensitivity of the method permits weighing of collected particles in less than 1 minute.

Beta Adsorption. Beta particles are adsorbed by dust particles deposited between the emitter and detector. Again, sensitivity is sufficient to permit less-than-one-minute measurement in concentrations under 1 mg/m^3 with typical cyclone flow rates.

Electrostatic Charge. When the charge on particles is allowed to drain off through an electrometer, the current flow is related to some parameter of the particles deposited. The relationship between the measurement obtained and the mass of respirable dust needs to be determined.

In addition to measuring the concentration of respirable coal mine dust, some work is being done to develop instruments to evaluate the size-distribution parameters of in-mine dust clouds. A mass distribution measuring instrument using a number of cyclones in parallel may permit cascade impactor-type measurements without their usual drawbacks. Laser beam scanning is being developed as a means of measuring both particle size and concentration.

Coal Mine Respirator Research

Aside from escape-type devices, the use of respirators in coal mines is not general. Investigations are underway to determine where and to what extent they are used and why they are not used where they would be appropriate. The effectiveness (protection factor) actually obtained when a respirator is used in typical mining operations will also be measured. These investigations will lead to work on the development of respirators for use in coal mines and the development of guidelines and criteria for their approval and use.

REFERENCES

1. Lippmann, M. (1970). *Amer. Ind. Hyg. Ass. J.* **31**, 138.
2. Lippmann, M., and Harris, W. B. (1962). *Health Phys.* **8**, 155.
3. Hatch, T. F., and Gross, P. (1964). "Pulmonary Deposition and Retention of Inhaled Aerosols." Academic, New York.
4. Orenstein, A. J., (Ed.). (1960). "Proceedings of the Pneumoconiosis Conference, Johannesburg, 1959." Churchill, London.